FEDERAL PHARMACY LAW EXAM PREP

By

Mark Thompson

This publication is for informational use only.

This publication is not intended to give legal advice. For legal advice, consult a legal professional.

This publication is not intended to diagnose, treat, or be construed as medical advice in any way.

Application of any information remains the professional responsibility of the practitioner.

The author does not assume and hereby disclaims any liability to any party for any loss, damage, and/or failure resulting from an error or omission, regardless of cause.

Table of Contents

SECTION I: FEDERAL PHARMACY LAW QUESTIONS AND ANSWERS

1. FEDERAL PHARMACY LAW QUESTIONS PART-1

1. Which federal agency oversees the regulation of controlled substances in the United States?

    a. FDA

    b. DEA

    c. CDC

    d. NIH

2. How many federal controlled substance schedules are there in the United States?

    a. 2

    b. 3

    c. 4

    d. 5

3. Which schedule includes drugs with the highest potential for abuse and no accepted medical use?

    a. Schedule I

    b. Schedule II

    c. Schedule III

    d. Schedule IV

4. Which schedule includes drugs with a high potential for abuse, accepted medical use, and severe restrictions on prescription refills?

   a. Schedule I

   b. Schedule II

   c. Schedule III

   d. Schedule IV

5. Which of the following is an example of a Schedule III controlled substance?

   a. Heroin

   b. Morphine

   c. Codeine

   d. Diazepam (Valium)

6. How often must pharmacies conduct an inventory of controlled substances?

   a. Monthly

   b. Quarterly

   c. Annually

   d. Biennially

7. Which federal form is used for ordering Schedule II controlled substances?

   a. DEA Form 106

   b. DEA Form 222

   c. DEA Form 41

   d. DEA Form 224

8. Which schedule includes drugs with a low potential for abuse and widely accepted medical use?

   a. Schedule I

   b. Schedule II

   c. Schedule III

   d. Schedule IV

9. What information must be included on a prescription for a Schedule II controlled substance?

   a. Patient's name and address

   b. Drug name, strength, and quantity

   c. Prescriber's DEA number

   d. All of the above

10. Which schedule includes drugs with a moderate potential for abuse and accepted medical use?

   a. Schedule I

   b. Schedule II

   c. Schedule III

   d. Schedule IV

11. Which schedule includes drugs with a low potential for abuse and accepted medical use but may lead to limited physical or psychological dependence?

   a. Schedule I

   b. Schedule II

   c. Schedule III

   d. Schedule IV

12. Which of the following is an example of a Schedule V controlled substance?

   a. Fentanyl

   b. Oxycodone

   c. Lisdexamfetamine (Vyvanse)

   d. Robitussin AC

13. Which DEA registration form is required for pharmacies that handle controlled substances?

    a. DEA Form 222

    b. DEA Form 224

    c. DEA Form 106

    d. DEA Form 41

14. Which schedule includes drugs with a very low potential for abuse and are primarily used for antidiarrheal, antitussive, and analgesic purposes?

    a. Schedule I

    b. Schedule II

    c. Schedule III

    d. Schedule V

15. Which of the following is NOT a requirement for a prescription of a Schedule II controlled substance?

    a. Electronic prescribing

    b. Handwritten prescription on an official prescription pad

    c. No refills allowed

    d. Prescriber's signature

16. How long must a pharmacy retain records related to the receipt and dispensing of controlled substances?

a. 1 year

b. 2 years

c. 3 years

d. 5 years

17. Which schedule includes drugs that are exempt from most of the controlled substance regulations and are typically available over-the-counter?

a. Schedule I

b. Schedule II

c. Schedule III

d. Schedule V

18. In the federal scheduling system, which schedule represents the highest level of control?

a. Schedule I

b. Schedule II

c. Schedule III

d. Schedule IV

19. Which schedule includes anabolic steroids and certain depressants and stimulants?

a. Schedule I

b. Schedule II

c. Schedule III

d. Schedule IV

20. What is the primary purpose of the federal controlled substances scheduling system?

a. To restrict access to prescription medications

b. To generate revenue for the DEA

c. To classify drugs based on their potential for abuse and medical use

d. To regulate the sale of over-the-counter drugs

21. Which federal agency oversees the regulation of controlled substances in the United States?

a. FDA

b. DEA

c. CDC

d. NIH

22. How many federal controlled substance schedules are there in the United States?

a. 2

b. 3

c. 4

d. 5

23 .Which schedule includes drugs with the highest potential for abuse and no accepted medical use?

a. Schedule I

b. Schedule II

c. Schedule III

d. Schedule IV

24. Which schedule includes drugs with a high potential for abuse, accepted medical use, and severe restrictions on prescription refills?

a. Schedule I

b. Schedule II

c. Schedule III

d. Schedule IV

25. Which of the following is an example of a Schedule III controlled substance?

a. Heroin

b. Morphine

c. Codeine

d. Diazepam (Valium)

26. How often must pharmacies conduct an inventory of controlled substances?

a. Monthly

b. Quarterly

c. Annually

d. Biennially

27. Which federal form is used for ordering Schedule II controlled substances?

a. DEA Form 106

b. DEA Form 222

c. DEA Form 41

d. DEA Form 224

28. Which schedule includes drugs with a low potential for abuse and widely accepted medical use?

a. Schedule I

b. Schedule II

c. Schedule III

d. Schedule IV2

29. What information must be included on a prescription for a Schedule II controlled substance?

a. Patient's name and address

b. Drug name, strength, and quantity

c. Prescriber's DEA number

d. All of the above

30. Which schedule includes drugs with a moderate potential for abuse and accepted medical use?

a. Schedule I

b. Schedule II

c. Schedule III

d. Schedule IV

31. Which schedule includes drugs with a low potential for abuse and accepted medical use but may lead to limited physical or psychological dependence?

a. Schedule I

b. Schedule II

c. Schedule III

d. Schedule IV

32. Which of the following is an example of a Schedule V controlled substance?

a. Fentanyl

b. Oxycodone

c. Lisdexamfetamine (Vyvanse)

d. Robitussin AC

33. Which DEA registration form is required for pharmacies that handle controlled substances?

a. DEA Form 222

b. DEA Form 224

c. DEA Form 106

d. DEA Form 41

34. Which schedule includes drugs with a very low potential for abuse and are primarily used for antidiarrheal, antitussive, and analgesic purposes?

a. Schedule I

b. Schedule II

c. Schedule III

d. Schedule V

35. Which of the following is NOT a requirement for a prescription of a Schedule II controlled substance?

a. Electronic prescribing

b. Handwritten prescription on an official prescription pad

c. No refills allowed

d. Prescriber's signature

36. How long must a pharmacy retain records related to the receipt and dispensing of controlled substances?

a. 1 year

b. 2 years

c. 3 years

d. 5 years

37. Which schedule includes drugs that are exempt from most of the controlled substance regulations and are typically available over-the-counter?

a. Schedule I

b. Schedule II

c. Schedule III

d. Schedule V

38. In the federal scheduling system, which schedule represents the highest level of control?

a. Schedule I

b. Schedule II

c. Schedule III

d. Schedule IV

39. Which schedule includes anabolic steroids and certain depressants and stimulants?

a. Schedule I

b. Schedule II

c. Schedule III

d. Schedule IV

40. What is the primary purpose of the federal controlled substances scheduling system?

a. To restrict access to prescription medications

b. To generate revenue for the DEA

c. To classify drugs based on their potential for abuse and medical use

d. To regulate the sale of over-the-counter drugs

41. Which federal agency oversees and enforces regulations related to pharmacy prescriptions in the United States?

a. FDA

b. DEA

c. CDC

d. NIH

42. What information must be included on a prescription for a controlled substance?

a. Patient's name and address

b. Prescriber's name, address, and DEA number

c. Medication name, strength, and quantity

d. All of the above

43. Which schedule of controlled substances requires a prescription to be handwritten, signed, and dated by the prescriber?

    a. Schedule I

    b. Schedule II

    c. Schedule III

    d. Schedule IV

44. How long is a prescription for a Schedule II controlled substance typically valid before it expires?

    a. 7 days

    b. 14 days

    c. 30 days

    d. 90 days

45. Which prescription refill category allows for the maximum number of refills without the need for a new prescription?

    a. Zero refills

    b. One refill

    c. Five refills

    d. Unlimited refills

46. What is the maximum duration for a Schedule III to V controlled substance prescription, including refills?

a. 7 days

b. 14 days

c. 30 days

d. 180 days

47. Which of the following prescription forms is required for controlled substances?

a. Standard prescription pad

b. Pre-printed prescription form

c. Tamper-resistant prescription form

d. E-prescription only

48. Who is authorized to issue a prescription for a controlled substance?

a. Any healthcare provider

b. Any licensed pharmacist

c. Only medical doctors (MDs)

d. Only pharmacists-in-charge

49. What is the federal law regarding the transfer of Schedule III to V controlled substance prescriptions between pharmacies?

   a. Transfer is not allowed.

   b. Transfers are allowed once.

   c. Transfers are allowed only within the same state.

   d. Transfers are allowed as many times as needed.

50. What must be included on the label of a dispensed prescription medication?

   a. Patient's home address

   b. Medication's generic name

   c. Manufacturer's phone number

   d. Pharmacist's signature

51. How often should pharmacies conduct an inventory of controlled substances?

   a. Weekly

   b. Monthly

   c. Annually

   d. Biennially

52. What is the maximum quantity of pseudoephedrine-containing products that an individual can purchase without a prescription in a single day?

   a. 7.5 grams

   b. 15 grams

   c. 30 grams

   d. 60 grams

53. Which federal law requires pharmacists to offer counseling to patients when they pick up new prescriptions?

   a. Controlled Substances Act

   b. Federal Food, Drug, and Cosmetic Act

   c. Drug Listing Act

   d. Omnibus Budget Reconciliation Act (OBRA) '90

54. What must be included in a medication profile for each patient at a pharmacy?

   a. Patient's email address

   b. Patient's social security number

   c. List of all medications dispensed to the patient

   d. Pharmacist's contact information

55. Which federal agency is responsible for regulating the labeling and packaging of prescription drugs?

a. DEA

b. CDC

c. FDA

d. NIH

56. Under federal law, how long must pharmacies retain prescription records?

a. 1 year

b. 2 years

c. 3 years

d. 5 years

57. What is the primary purpose of federal prescription requirements?

a. To generate revenue for the government

b. To simplify the prescription process for patients

c. To ensure the safe and effective use of prescription medications

d. To restrict access to prescription medications

58. Which of the following is NOT typically required on a prescription label?

a. Patient's date of birth

b. Medication name and strength

c. Dosage instructions

d. Refill information

59. What is the federal requirement for the storage of prescription records?

a. Must be stored off-site

b. Must be stored in a secure and retrievable manner

c. Must be kept indefinitely

d. Must be stored with patient records

60. What is the purpose of requiring tamper-resistant prescription paper for certain controlled substances?

a. To prevent counterfeiting of prescriptions

b. To reduce the cost of prescription paper

c. To make prescriptions easier to read

d. To encourage electronic prescribing

61. What is the primary role of a pharmacist in a federal pharmacy setting?

a. Diagnosing medical conditions

b. Dispensing medications

c. Performing surgery

d. Conducting research

62. Which federal agency sets the standards and regulations for the practice of pharmacy in the United States?

a. FDA (Food and Drug Administration)

b. DEA (Drug Enforcement Administration)

c. CDC (Centers for Disease Control and Prevention)

d. NABP (National Association of Boards of Pharmacy)

63. What is the primary responsibility of a pharmacist regarding prescription medications?

a. Diagnosing medical conditions

b. Monitoring patient vital signs

c. Ensuring the safe and effective use of medications

d. Filling out insurance claims

64. In a federal pharmacy, what is the pharmacist's role in verifying prescriptions?

   a. Counting pills

   b. Ensuring the prescription is valid and appropriate

   c. Writing the prescription

   d. Administering the medication

65. Which federal law requires pharmacists to offer counseling to patients when they receive new prescriptions?

   a. Drug Enforcement Act

   b. Food, Drug, and Cosmetic Act

   c. Omnibus Budget Reconciliation Act (OBRA) '90

   d. Controlled Substances Act

66. What is the pharmacist's responsibility regarding prescription drug storage in a pharmacy?

   a. Setting prices for medications

   b. Monitoring inventory levels

   c. Ensuring proper storage conditions

   d. Administering vaccines

67. Which of the following is NOT a duty typically performed by pharmacists in a federal pharmacy setting?

a. Compounding medications

b. Conducting medical surgeries

c. Drug utilization review

d. Collaborating with healthcare providers

68. What is the pharmacist's role in managing drug interactions and adverse effects?

a. Ignoring potential interactions

b. Dispensing medications without warnings

c. Providing information and counseling to patients

d. Keeping interactions confidential

69. What federal agency is responsible for enforcing laws related to controlled substances in pharmacies?

a. FDA

b. CDC

c. DEA

d. NIH

70. What is the pharmacist's role in addressing medication non-adherence by patients?

a. Blaming the patient for non-adherence

b. Refusing to dispense medications

c. Identifying reasons for non-adherence and providing solutions

d. Reporting non-adherent patients to the police

71. How can pharmacists contribute to public health initiatives in federal pharmacy settings?

a. By advocating for the use of unproven alternative medicines

b. By discouraging vaccination

c. By providing immunization services and health education

d. By promoting medication non-adherence

72. What role do pharmacists play in medication therapy management (MTM)?

a. They don't have any role in MTM.

b. They provide MTM services to optimize medication use.

c. They only dispense medications without providing counseling.

d. They write prescriptions for patients.

73. In a federal pharmacy, what is the pharmacist's responsibility when a patient presents a prescription with unclear or illegible instructions?

a. Dispense the medication as-is

b. Guess what the prescriber intended

c. Contact the prescriber to clarify the instructions

d. Refuse to fill the prescription

74. What is the pharmacist's role in ensuring patient privacy and confidentiality in federal pharmacy settings?

a. Sharing patient information with anyone who asks

b. Encrypting patient data for security

c. Keeping patient information confidential and secure

d. Posting patient information online

75. What federal agency is responsible for regulating the labeling and packaging of prescription drugs?

a. DEA

b. CDC

c. FDA

d. NABP

76. In a federal pharmacy, what is the pharmacist's responsibility when a medication recall is issued by the manufacturer?

a. Ignore the recall and continue dispensing the medication

b. Notify the patients and return the recalled medication to the manufacturer

c. Keep the recalled medication in stock for future use

d. Dispose of the recalled medication in regular trash

77. How often should pharmacists conduct medication therapy reviews for patients in a federal pharmacy setting?

a. Monthly

b. Quarterly

c. Annually

d. As needed

78. What is the pharmacist's role in providing patient education regarding prescription medications?

a. Withholding information from patients

b. Explaining medication usage, side effects, and potential interactions

c. Recommending over-the-counter alternatives

d. Providing medical diagnoses

79. How can pharmacists contribute to the prevention of prescription drug abuse in a federal pharmacy setting?

   a. Dispensing controlled substances without question

   b. Monitoring patient activities

   c. Refusing to fill any controlled substance prescriptions

   d. Educating patients about the risks of prescription drug abuse

80. In a federal pharmacy, what should a pharmacist do if they suspect prescription forgery or fraud?

   a. Ignore the suspicion

   b. Report it to the local news media

   c. Report it to the appropriate authorities and document the suspicion

   d. Confront the patient directly

81. What is compounding in the context of pharmacy practice?

   a. The preparation of prescription medications by pharmaceutical manufacturers

   b. The practice of mixing different commercially available medications

   c. The customization of medications for individual patients

   d. The process of repackaging over-the-counter drugs

82. Which federal agency regulates compounding pharmacies in the United States?

a. FDA (Food and Drug Administration)

b. DEA (Drug Enforcement Administration)

c. CDC (Centers for Disease Control and Prevention)

d. NIH (National Institutes of Health)

83. Under what conditions can a compounding pharmacy produce large quantities of compounded medications without individual prescriptions?

a. Always, as long as the pharmacy is licensed

b. Only for medications on the FDA's Drug Shortage List

c. Only with a waiver from the DEA

d. Never, unless there's a patient-specific prescription

84. What is the purpose of the Drug Quality and Security Act (DQSA) in relation to compounding?

a. It bans all compounding practices in the United States.

b. It establishes a clear distinction between traditional compounding and outsourcing facilities.

c. It requires pharmacists to obtain a separate license for compounding.

d. It allows compounding without any federal oversight.

85. When can a compounding pharmacy compound a medication that is essentially a copy of an FDA-approved commercially available drug?

a. Always, to meet patient preferences

b. Only if the patient requests it specifically

c. Only when there is a documented drug shortage

d. Never, it's not allowed

86. What is a 503B outsourcing facility in the context of compounding?

a. A pharmacy that specializes in compounding for individual patients

b. A pharmacy that does not require FDA registration

c. A facility that compounds large quantities of medications and is subject to federal oversight

d. A facility that can compound medications without any restrictions

87. In compounding, what is the Beyond-Use Date (BUD)?

a. The date until which a medication is safe to use after compounding

b. The date until which a medication is effective

c. The date of manufacture

d. The expiration date on the original drug container

88. What is the purpose of the United States Pharmacopeia (USP) Chapter <797>?

a. To regulate the pricing of compounded medications

b. To establish quality standards for sterile compounding

c. To promote over-the-counter medications

d. To oversee drug manufacturing by pharmaceutical companies

89. Which of the following is a key component of aseptic compounding in pharmacy practice?

a. Handwashing before and after compounding

b. Using non-sterile equipment

c. Compounding in a non-sterile environment

d. Using expired ingredients

90. What is the purpose of compounding recordkeeping and documentation?

a. To justify charging higher prices for compounded medications

b. To track inventory for tax purposes

c. To demonstrate compliance with regulations and ensure traceability

d. To promote the pharmacy's branding

91. Which of the following statements about non-sterile compounding is true?

    a. It requires less attention to cleanliness compared to sterile compounding.

    b. It is never performed in community pharmacies.

    c. It involves preparing medications in a non-sterile environment.

    d. It is less regulated than sterile compounding.

92. What should pharmacists do if they discover that a compounded medication is contaminated or otherwise compromised?

    a. Sell it at a discounted price

    b. Dispose of it immediately

    c. Continue dispensing it and monitor patients for adverse effects

    d. Report it to the FDA

93. Which organization sets the standards for quality and safety in pharmaceutical compounding?

    a. DEA

    b. CDC

    c. USP

    d. NABP

94. What is the purpose of the Pharmacy Compounding Accreditation Board (PCAB)?

a. To provide accreditation for compounding pharmacies

b. To inspect compounding pharmacies for safety violations

c. To set drug pricing standards for compounded medications

d. To promote non-sterile compounding practices

95. What is the role of a pharmacist in ensuring the quality of raw materials used in compounding?

a. No responsibility; it's the supplier's responsibility

b. Verify the supplier's reputation and trust their claims

c. Conduct quality testing on each batch of raw materials

d. Reject any raw materials that appear substandard

96. What is the primary goal of compounding pharmacists when customizing medications for patients?

a. To increase the shelf life of medications

b. To reduce the cost of medications

c. To improve patient adherence and outcomes

d. To bypass the need for prescriptions

97. In compounding, what does "beyond-use date" (BUD) signify?

a. The date of manufacture

b. The date until which a medication is safe and effective

c. The date of FDA approval

d. The date of prescription

98. When might a pharmacist need to compound a medication due to patient allergies or sensitivities?

a. When the patient requests it for convenience

b. When the patient prefers the taste of a compounded version

c. When the commercially available form contains allergenic ingredients

d. When the pharmacist wants to charge higher prices

99. Which of the following is NOT a principle of good compounding practice?

a. Ensuring appropriate labeling

b. Preparing medications in a non-sterile environment

c. Documenting the compounding process

d. Maintaining proper hygiene and cleanliness

1. FEDERAL PHARMACY LAW ANSWERS PART-1

1. Answer: B

DEA (Drug Enforcement Administration).

Explanation: The DEA is responsible for enforcing the Controlled Substances Act and regulating Controlled substances in the U.S.

2. Answer: D

5.

Explanation: Controlled substances are categorized into five schedules (Schedule I-V) based on their Potential for abuse and medical use.

3. Answer: A

Schedule I.

Explanation: Schedule I drugs have a high potential for abuse and no accepted medical use in the United States.

4. Answer: B

Schedule II.

Explanation: Schedule II drugs have a high potential for abuse, accepted medical use, but are subject to strict regulations, including no refills without a new prescription.

5. Answer: D

Diazepam (Valium).

Explanation: Diazepam is a Schedule IV controlled substance, not Schedule III.

6. Answer: C

Annually

Explanation: Federal law requires pharmacies to conduct an annual inventory of controlled substances.

7. Answer: B

DEA Form 222.

Explanation: DEA Form 222 is used to order Schedule II controlled substances.

8. Answer: D

Schedule IV.

Explanation: Schedule IV drugs have a low potential for abuse and accepted medical uses.

9. Answer: D

All of the above.

Explanation: A prescription for a Schedule II controlled substance must include all of these elements.

10. Answer: C

Schedule III.

Explanation: Schedule III drugs have a moderate potential for abuse and accepted medical uses.

11. **Answer: D**

Schedule IV.

Explanation: Schedule IV drugs have a low potential for abuse and accepted medical uses but may lead to limited physical or psychological dependence.

12. **Answer: D**

Robitussin AC.

Explanation: Robitussin AC is an example of a Schedule V controlled substance.

13. **Answer: B**

DEA Form 224.

Explanation: DEA Form 224 is used for pharmacy registration to handle controlled substances.

14. **Answer: D**

Schedule V.

Explanation: Schedule V drugs have a very low potential for abuse and are primarily used for antidiarrheal, antitussive, and analgesic purposes.

15. **Answer: A**

Electronic prescribing.

Explanation: Electronic prescribing is allowed for Schedule II controlled substances in some states, provided certain conditions are met.

16. **Answer: D**

5 years.

Explanation: Pharmacies must retain records related to the receipt and dispensing of controlled substances for at least 5 years.

17. **Answer: D**

Schedule V.

Explanation: Schedule V drugs are exempt from most of the controlled substance regulations and are typically available over- the-counter.

18. **Answer: A**

Schedule I.

Explanation: Schedule I represents the highest level of control due to the high potential for abuse and lack of accepted medical use.

19. **Answer: B**

Schedule II.

Explanation: Schedule II includes anabolic steroids and certain depressants and stimulants.

20. **Answer: C**

To classify drugs based on their potential for abuse and medical use.

Explanation: The federal controlled substances scheduling system categorizes drugs based on their potential for abuse and accepted medical uses to regulate their handling and distribution.

21. Answer: B

DEA (Drug Enforcement Administration).

Explanation: The DEA is responsible for enforcing the Controlled Substances Act and regulating controlled substances in the U.S.

22. **Answer: D**

5.

Explanation: Controlled substances are categorized into five schedules (Schedule I-V) based on their Potential for abuse and medical use.

23. **Answer: A**

Schedule I.

Explanation: Schedule I drugs have a high potential for abuse and no accepted medical use in the United States.

24. **Answer: B**

Schedule II.

Explanation: Schedule II drugs have a high potential for abuse, accepted medical use, but are subject to strict regulations, including no refills without a new prescription.

25. **Answer: D**

Diazepam (Valium).

Explanation: Diazepam is a Schedule IV controlled substance, not Schedule III.

26. **Answer: C**

Annually.

Explanation: Federal law requires pharmacies to conduct an annual inventory of controlled substances.

27. **Answer: B**

DEA Form 222.

Explanation: DEA Form 222 is used to order Schedule II controlled substances.

28. **Answer: D**

Schedule IV.

Explanation: Schedule IV drugs have a low potential for abuse and accepted medical uses.

29. **Answer: D**

All of the above.

Explanation: A prescription for a Schedule II controlled substance must include all of these elements.

30. **Answer: C**

Schedule III.

Explanation: Schedule III drugs have a moderate potential for abuse and accepted medical uses.

31. **Answer: D**

Schedule IV.

Explanation: Schedule IV drugs have a low potential for abuse and accepted medical uses but may lead to limited physical or psychological dependence.

32. **Answer: D**

Robitussin AC.

Explanation: Robitussin AC is an example of a Schedule V controlled substance.

33. **Answer: B**

DEA Form 224.

Explanation: DEA Form 224 is used for pharmacy registration to handle controlled substances.

34. **Answer: D**

Schedule V.

Explanation: Schedule V drugs have a very low potential for abuse and are primarily used for antidiarrheal, Antitussive, and analgesic purposes.

35. **Answer: A**

Electronic prescribing.

Explanation: Electronic prescribing is allowed for Schedule II controlled substances in some states, provided certain conditions are met.

36. **Answer: D**

5 years.

Explanation: Pharmacies must retain records related to the receipt and dispensing of controlled substances for at least 5 years.

37. **Answer: D**

Schedule V.

Explanation: Schedule V drugs are exempt from most of the controlled substance regulations and are typically available over-the-counter.

38. **Answer: A**

Schedule I.

Explanation: Schedule I represents the highest level of control due to the high potential for abuse and lack of accepted medical use.

39. **Answer: B**

Schedule II.

Explanation: Schedule II includes anabolic steroids and certain depressants and stimulants.

40. **Answer: C**

To classify drugs based on their potential for abuse and medical use.

Explanation: The federal controlled substances scheduling system categorizes drugs based on their potential for abuse and accepted medical uses to regulate their handling and distribution.

41. **Answer: B**

DEA (Drug Enforcement Administration).

Explanation: The DEA plays a significant role in enforcing federal prescription regulations.

42. **Answer: D**

All of the above.

Explanation: A prescription for a controlled substance must include all these elements.

43. **Answer: B**

Schedule II.

Explanation: Schedule II prescriptions must be handwritten, signed, and dated by the prescriber.

44. **Answer: B**

14 days.

Explanation: Most Schedule II prescriptions are valid for 14 days from the date of issuance.

45. **Answer: A**

Zero refills.

Explanation: Schedule II prescriptions typically allow for zero refills.

46. **Answer: D**

180 days.

Explanation: Schedule III to V controlled substance prescriptions, including refills, are typically valid for up to 180 days.

47. **Answer: C**

Tamper-resistant prescription form.

Explanation: Controlled substance prescriptions must be written on tamper-resistant paper or electronic formats that meet specific security criteria.

48. **Answer: C**

Explanation: Only medical doctors (MDs) and other authorized healthcare providers can issue prescriptions for controlled substances.

49. **Answer: B**

Transfers are allowed once between pharmacies.

Explanation: Certain conditions must be met, and the pharmacies involved must record the transfer.

50. **Answer: B**

Medication's generic name.

Explanation: The label on dispensed prescription medications should include the medication's generic name, among other information.

51. **Answer: C**

Annually.

Explanation: Pharmacies are required to conduct an annual inventory of controlled substances.

52. **Answer: A**

7.5 grams.

Explanation: Federal regulations limit the purchase of pseudoephedrine-containing products to 7.5 grams per day and 30 grams per month per individual.

53. **Answer: D**

Omnibus Budget Reconciliation Act (OBRA) '90.

Explanation: OBRA '90 requires pharmacists to offer counseling to Medicaid patients when they receive new prescriptions.

54. **Answer: C**

List of all medications dispensed to the patient.

Explanation: A medication profile includes a record of all medications dispensed to a patient at the Pharmacy.

55. **Answer: C**

FDA (Food and Drug Administration).

Explanation: The FDA regulates the labeling and packaging of prescription drugs to ensure safety and efficacy.

56. **Answer: D**

5 years.

Explanation: Federal law requires pharmacies to retain prescription records for a minimum of 5 years.

57. **Answer: C**

To ensure the safe and effective use of prescription medications.

Explanation: Federal prescription requirements are primarily in place to safeguard patients and promote safe medication use.

58. **Answer: A**

Patient's date of birth.

Explanation: The patient's date of birth is not typically included on the prescription label.

59. **Answer: B**

Must be stored in a secure and retrievable manner.

Explanation: Prescription records must be stored securely and be easily retrievable for a specified period.

60. **Answer: A**

To prevent counterfeiting of prescriptions.

Explanation: Tamper-resistant prescription paper is designed to prevent the unauthorized duplication or alteration of prescriptions for controlled substances.

61. **Answer: B**

Dispensing medications.

Explanation: Pharmacists play a central role in ensuring the safe and accurate dispensing of medications in a pharmacy setting.

62. **Answer: D**

NABP (National Association of Boards of Pharmacy).

Explanation: While multiple federal agencies have roles in pharmacy regulations, NABP is responsible for setting standards for pharmacy practice.

63. **Answer: C**

Ensuring the safe and effective use of medications.

Explanation: Pharmacists are responsible for providing medication therapy management to ensure that medications are used safely and effectively.

64. **Answer: B**

Ensuring the prescription is valid and appropriate.

Explanation: Pharmacists must review prescriptions for accuracy, legality, and appropriateness before dispensing medication.

65. **Answer: C**

Omnibus Budget Reconciliation Act (OBRA) '90.

Explanation: OBRA '90 requires pharmacists to offer counseling to Medicaid patients receiving new prescriptions.

66. **Answer: C**

Ensuring proper storage conditions.

Explanation: Pharmacists are responsible for maintaining appropriate storage conditions to ensure the integrity and safety of medications.

67. **Answer: B**

Conducting medical surgeries.

Explanation: Pharmacists do not perform medical surgeries; their primary role is related to medication management and counseling.

68. **Answer: C**

Providing information and counseling to patients.

Explanation: Pharmacists are responsible for educating patients about potential drug interactions and adverse effects.

69. **Answer: C**

DEA (Drug Enforcement Administration).

Explanation: The DEA enforces laws related to controlled substances in pharmacies.

70. **Answer: C**

Identifying reasons for non-adherence and providing solutions.

Explanation: Pharmacists play a crucial role in helping patients overcome barriers to medication adherence.

71. **Answer: C**

By providing immunization services and health education.

Explanation: Pharmacists can contribute to public health by offering immunizations and health education to the community.

72. **Answer: B**

They provide MTM services to optimize medication use.

Explanation: Pharmacists are trained to offer MTM services to help patients achieve optimal medication therapy outcomes.

73. **Answer: C**

Contact the prescriber to clarify the instructions.

Explanation: Pharmacists should contact the prescriber to ensure the prescription is clear and appropriate For the patient.

74. **Answer: C**

Keeping patient information confidential and secure.

Explanation: Pharmacists must protect patient privacy and adhere to HIPAA regulations.

75. **Answer: C**

FDA (Food and Drug Administration).

Explanation: The FDA regulates the labeling and packaging of prescription drugs to ensure safety and effectiveness.

76. **Answer: B**

Notify the patients and return the recalled medication to the manufacturer.

Explanation: Pharmacists should follow proper procedures to address medication recalls.

77. **Answer: D**

As needed.

Explanation: Pharmacists should conduct medication therapy reviews as necessary based on patient needs and changes in therapy.

78. **Answer: B**

Explaining medication usage, side effects, and potential interactions.

Explanation: Pharmacists are responsible for providing comprehensive patient education on prescription medications.

79. **Answer: D**

Educating patients about the risks of prescription drug abuse.

Explanation: Pharmacists can play a role in preventing abuse by providing education and monitoring for potential signs of abuse.

80. **Answer: C**

Report it to the appropriate authorities and document the suspicion.

Explanation: Pharmacists should report suspected forgery or fraud to the appropriate law enforcement agencies and document the incident for their records.

81. **Answer: C**

The customization of medications for individual patients.

Explanation: Compounding involves preparing medications tailored to a patient's specific needs.

82. **Answer: A**

FDA (Food and Drug Administration).

Explanation: The FDA regulates compounding pharmacies to ensure safety and quality.

83. **Answer: B**

Only for medications on the FDA's Drug Shortage List.

Explanation: Compounding pharmacies can produce larger quantities without individual prescriptions when there is a drug shortage and it's on the FDA's list.

84. **Answer: B**

It establishes a clear distinction between traditional compounding and outsourcing facilities.

Explanation: DQSA provides a framework for differentiating between various compounding practices.

85. **Answer: C**

Only when there is a documented drug shortage.

Explanation: Compounding such medications is typically reserved for cases of drug shortages.

86. **Answer: C**

A facility that compounds large quantities of medications and is subject to federal oversight.

Explanation: 503B outsourcing facilities are subject to FDA regulations.

87. **Answer: A**

The date until which a medication is safe to use after compounding.

Explanation: BUD is based on stability data and indicates the safe use of the compounded medication.

88. **Answer: B**

To establish quality standards for sterile compounding.

Explanation: USP Chapter <797> provides guidelines for sterile compounding practices.

89. **Answer: A**

Handwashing before and after compounding.

Explanation: Maintaining aseptic conditions is crucial, including proper hand hygiene.

90. **Answer: C**

To demonstrate compliance with regulations and ensure traceability.

Explanation: Recordkeeping is essential for regulatory compliance and patient safety.

91. **Answer: C**

It involves preparing medications in a non-sterile environment.

Explanation: Non-sterile compounding still requires attention to cleanliness and is subject to regulations.

92. **Answer: B**

Dispose of it immediately.

Explanation: Pharmacists should not dispense compromised compounded medications and should follow proper disposal procedures.

93. **Answer: C**

NABP

USP (United States Pharmacopeia).

Explanation: USP sets the standards for quality and safety in pharmaceutical compounding through chapters like <797>.

94. **Answer: A**

To provide accreditation for compounding pharmacies.

Explanation: PCAB offers accreditation to compounding pharmacies meeting specific quality and safety standards.

95. **Answer: D**

Reject any raw materials that appear substandard.

Explanation: Pharmacists should ensure the quality of raw materials used in compounding.

96. **Answer: C**

To improve patient adherence and outcomes.

Explanation: Compounding aims to tailor medications to better meet individual patient needs.

97. **Answer: B**

The date until which a medication is safe and effective.

Explanation: BUD is a critical component of ensuring patient safety in compounding.

98. **Answer: C**

When the commercially available form contains allergenic ingredients.

Explanation: Compounding can help when a patient has allergies or sensitivities to specific ingredients in commercial medications.

99. **Answer: B**

Preparing medications in a non-sterile environment.

Explanation: Good compounding practices emphasize the importance of sterile and controlled environments for sterile compounding.

2. FEDERAL PHARMACY LAW QUESTIONS PART-2

1. What is the pharmacist's role in providing quality assurance for compounded medications?

   a. It is not the pharmacist's responsibility.

   b. Conducting random inspections of the compounding area

   c. Ensuring compliance with USP standards and performing quality checks

   d. Reviewing marketing strategies for compounded medications

2. What is the primary purpose of classifying controlled substances into different schedules, including Class II?

   a. To categorize drugs based on their potential for abuse and accepted medical use

   b. To set drug prices in the market

   c. To limit access to certain medications

   d. To regulate the sale of over-the-counter drugs

3. Which federal agency is responsible for overseeing the scheduling of controlled substances in the United States?

   a. FDA (Food and Drug Administration)

   b. CDC (Centers for Disease Control and Prevention)

   c. DEA (Drug Enforcement Administration)

   d. NIH (National Institutes of Health)

4. Which of the following drugs is typically classified as a Class II controlled substance?

   a. Antibiotics

   b. Over-the-counter pain relievers

   c. Methadone

   d. Vitamins

5. What is the key characteristic of Class II controlled substances that distinguishes them from other schedules?

   a. They have a high potential for abuse.

   b. They are available without a prescription.

   c. They can be refilled multiple times.

   d. They are not subject to federal regulations.

6. How often can a prescription for a Class II controlled substance typically be refilled?

   a. As many times as the patient requests

   b. Once, within 72 hours of the original prescription

   c. Never, refills are not allowed

   d. Up to five times within six months

7. What is required on a prescription for a Class II controlled substance to make it valid and legal?

a. Only the patient's name

b. Only the prescriber's DEA number

c. The patient's name, prescriber's signature, and drug name

d. The pharmacist's signature

8. In the event of theft or loss of a controlled substance, what must a pharmacy do to comply with federal law?

a. Report the incident to the local police department

b. Notify the DEA within one business day

c. Dispose of all controlled substances in the pharmacy

d. Ignore the incident, as it's a common occurrence

9. How often must pharmacies conduct an inventory of Class II controlled substances?

a. Weekly

b. Monthly

c. Annually

d. Biennially

10. What is the federal law regarding the transfer of Class II controlled substance prescriptions between pharmacies?

a. Transfer is not allowed.

b. Transfers are allowed once.

c. Transfers are allowed only within the same state.

d. Transfers are allowed as many times as needed.

11. Which of the following is NOT a requirement for filling a prescription for a Class II controlled substance?

a. The prescription must be written on tamper-resistant paper.

b. The pharmacist must record the prescription in a central database.

c. The pharmacist must verify the prescriber's DEA number.

d. The patient must provide valid identification.

12. What is the federal requirement for the storage of prescription records for Class II controlled substances?

a. Must be stored off-site

b. Must be stored in a secure and retrievable manner

c. Must be kept indefinitely

d. Must be shredded after one year

13. How does the federal government classify substances into different schedules, including Class II?

    a. Based solely on their medical use

    b. Based solely on their potential for abuse

    c. Based on a combination of their potential for abuse and medical use

    d. Based on their cost and availability

14. What is the primary purpose of federal regulations surrounding Class II controlled substances?

    a. To generate revenue for the government

    b. To simplify the prescription process for patients

    c. To ensure the safe and secure handling of these substances

    d. To restrict access to necessary medications

15. What information must be included on the label of a dispensed prescription for a Class II controlled substance?

    a. Patient's date of birth

    b. Medication's generic name

    c. Dosage instructions

    d. Refill information

16. What is the role of a pharmacist in verifying the legitimacy of a Class II controlled substance prescription?

a. Accept all prescriptions without question

b. Verify the patient's insurance coverage first

c. Ensure the prescription is valid, including the prescriber's DEA number and patient information

d. Call the patient to confirm their identity

17. What is the federal law regarding the storage of Class II controlled substances in a pharmacy?

a. They must be stored in unlocked cabinets for easy access.

b. They must be stored separately from other medications in a locked cabinet or safe.

c. They can be stored with non-controlled substances.

d. They must be stored openly on pharmacy shelves.

18. In which federal schedule are medications with the lowest potential for abuse categorized?

a. Schedule I

b. Schedule II

c. Schedule III

d. Schedule V

19. What is the federal requirement for documenting the transfer of a Class II controlled substance prescription?

    a. No documentation is needed.

    b. A record of the transfer must be maintained at the transferring pharmacy only.

    c. Both the transferring and receiving pharmacies must maintain records of the transfer.

    d. The patient must sign a waiver for the transfer.

20. What is the purpose of the "closed system" for Class II controlled substances?

    a. To restrict access to these substances to a select group of healthcare providers

    b. To prevent the diversion and abuse of these substances

    c. To allow over-the-counter sales of Class II substances

    d. To eliminate the need for prescription requirements

21. How do federal laws regarding Class II controlled substances impact the practice of telepharmacy?

    a. Tele pharmacy is not allowed for Class II substances.

    b. Tele pharmacy is only allowed for Class II refills.

    c. Tele pharmacy is allowed for Class II prescriptions under specific conditions.

    d. Tele pharmacy is exempt from federal regulations.

22. What is misbranding in the context of Federal pharmacy law?

    a. Mixing different medications in the same container

    b. Marketing a generic drug without FDA approval

    c. Providing false or misleading labeling or advertising for a drug

    d. Selling prescription medications without a valid prescription

23. What is the primary purpose of drug labeling according to Federal pharmacy law?

    a. To provide marketing information to healthcare professionals

    b. To make the medication look appealing to patients

    c. To educate patients about the drug's risks and benefits

    d. To increase the price of the medication

24. Which federal agency is responsible for enforcing regulations related to drug labeling and misbranding?

    a. CDC (Centers for Disease Control and Prevention)

    b. DEA (Drug Enforcement Administration)

    c. FDA (Food and Drug Administration)

    d. NIH (National Institutes of Health)

25. What does it mean for a drug to be considered adulterated under Federal pharmacy law?

    a. The drug is counterfeit.

    b. The drug contains an approved ingredient in an incorrect quantity.

    c. The drug is not stored at the correct temperature.

    d. The drug is contaminated or unsafe for use.

26. Which of the following situations would NOT typically lead to a drug being considered adulterated?

    a. Contamination with harmful bacteria during manufacturing

    b. Failure to meet FDA requirements for strength and purity

    c. Having a label that is difficult to read

    d. Misrepresentation of the drug's ingredients on the label

27. What is the primary responsibility of pharmacists regarding misbranded or adulterated drugs in their inventory?

    a. To sell them to consumers at discounted prices

    b. To notify the FDA about the issue27.

    c. To dispose of them immediately

    d. To continue dispensing them with proper warnings

28. Which type of labeling is required for over-the-counter (OTC) drugs to help consumers use them safely?

    a. Prescription labels

    b. Child-resistant packaging

    c. Drug facts labeling

    d. Expiration date labeling

29. What does the "Rx Only" label on a medication mean?

    a. The medication can only be dispensed with a prescription.

    b. The medication is intended for use by healthcare professionals only.

    c. The medication is not approved by the FDA.

    d. The medication is available without a prescription.

30. Under Federal pharmacy law, what is the role of pharmacists in ensuring that prescription drug labeling is accurate and compliant?

    a. It is not the respon27sibility of pharmacists.

    b. To create their own labels for prescriptions

    c. To verify the accuracy of prescription labels and make corrections if necessary

    d. To report labeling issues to the patient's insurance company

31. What is the primary purpose of the Drug Listing Act in relation to drug labeling?

a. To establish pricing guidelines for prescription drugs

b. To require pharmacies to list their drug inventory online

c. To create a database of all drugs in commercial distribution

d. To ban the advertising of prescription medications

32. What federal agency is primarily responsible for regulating the manufacturing and distribution of prescription drugs in the United States?

a. FDA

b. DEA

c. CDC

d. CMS

33. Which federal law requires pharmacies to maintain patient privacy and confidentiality of medical records?

a. FDCA

b. HIPAA

c. DEA

d. ACA

34. Under federal law, which schedule of controlled substances has the highest potential for abuse?

a. 33. Schedule I

b. Schedule II

c. Schedule III

d. Schedule IV

35. Which federal agency enforces laws related to the controlled substances scheduling and registration of prescribers and pharmacies?

a. FDA

b. DEA

c. CMS

d. CDC

36. The Orange Book is a publication by the FDA that provides information about:

a. Over-the-counter drugs

b. Generic drug approvals

c. Drug recalls

d. Drug pricing

37. Which federal law requires pharmacies to offer counseling to Medicaid patients and maintain policies for drug utilization review?

a. HIPAA

b. FDCA

c. OBRA '90

d. CSA

38. Which federal law regulates the compounding of medications by pharmacies and outsourcing facilities?

a. FDCA

b. DSHEA

c. FDAAA

d. DQSA

39. The Drug Supply Chain Security Act (DSCSA) primarily addresses:

a. Drug advertising

b. Drug recalls

c. Drug importation

d. Drug traceability

40. Which federal law established the FDA's authority to regulate the marketing and promotion of prescription drugs?

 a. Kefauver-Harris Amendment

 b. Hatch-Waxman Act

 c. Durham-Humphrey Amendment

 d. Prescription Drug User Fee Act (PDUFA)

41. What is the maximum refills allowed for a Schedule III controlled substance prescription under federal law?

 a. 0 refills

 b. 1 refill

 c. 5 refills

 d. Unlimited refills

42. Which federal law established the National Provider Identifier (NPI) and requires healthcare providers, including pharmacists, to obtain one?

 a. HIPAA

 b. FDCA

 c. ACA

 d. DQSA

43. The Federal Food, Drug, and Cosmetic Act (FDCA) primarily focuses on:

a. Drug scheduling

b. Drug safety and efficacy

c. Drug pricing

d. Drug importation

44. Which federal law requires pharmacies to offer to counsel on the use of prescription medications to all patients?

a. HIPAA

b. FDCA

c. CSA

d. OBRA '90

45. The federal law that created the Drug Enforcement Administration (DEA) is:

a. CSA

b. FDCA

c. DSCSA

d. HIPAA

46. Which federal agency is responsible for regulating and overseeing clinical trials for new drugs?

a. FDA

b. CDC

c. NIH

d. DEA

47. The Drug Price Competition and Patent Term Restoration Act, commonly known as the Hatch-Waxman Act, primarily addresses:

a. Drug pricing

b. Generic drug approval

c. Drug importation

d. Drug recalls

48. Which of the following is a requirement of the Ryan Haight Online Pharmacy Consumer Protection Act?

a. Registration of online pharmacies with the DEA

b. Mandatory counseling for all online prescription orders

c. A ban on online pharmacies

d. Mandatory background checks for online pharmacy customers

49. Which federal agency enforces laws related to dietary supplements?

   a. FDA

   b. DEA48

   c. CDC

   d. FTC

50. The Federal Anti-Tampering Act primarily addresses:

   a. Drug importation

   b. Drug recalls

   c. Product tampering of consumer goods

   d. Drug pricing

51. Which federal agency is responsible for regulating the labeling and advertising of over-the-counter (OTC) drugs?

   a. FDA

   b. DEA

   c. CDC

   d. FTC

52. The Drug Quality and Security Act (DQSA) was enacted in response to concerns about:

a. Counterfeit drugs

b. Drug pricing51.

c. Prescription drug abuse

d. Drug recalls

53. Which federal law established the Prescription Drug Monitoring Program (PDMP) to track controlled substance prescriptions?

a. CSA

b. FDCA

c. DSCSA

d. DQSA

54. What is the maximum allowed quantity of pseudoephedrine-containing products that can be sold to an individual in a single day without a prescription under federal law?

a. 3.6 grams

b. 7.5 grams

c. 9 grams

d. 12 grams

55. Which federal agency regulates the labeling and advertising of prescription drugs?

a. DEA

b. FTC

c. FDA

d. CDC

56. The Dietary Supplement Health and Education Act (DSHEA) primarily:

a. Regulates dietary supplements as drugs

b. Regulates dietary supplement manufacturing

c. Requires dietary supplement prescriptions

d. Bans dietary supplements

57. Which federal law established a framework for the approval and regulation of biosimilars in the United States?

a. DSCSA

b. BPCI Act

c. Hatch-Waxman Act57.

d. FDCA

58. The Orphan Drug Act provides incentives for the development of drugs for rare diseases. What is the designation given to such drugs?

   a. Priority Review

   b. Orphan Drug Designation

   c. Accelerated Approval

   d. Breakthrough Therapy

59. Under the Drug Supply Chain Security Act (DSCSA), which entity is required to provide product tracing information when a prescription drug product is transferred?

   a. Manufacturer

   b. Wholesaler

   c. Pharmacy

   d. Patient

60. Which federal law allows patients to request access to their own medical records and requires healthcare providers to provide them with a copy?

   a. HIPAA

   b. FDCA

   c. DSCSA

   d. BPCI Act

61. Which of the following is NOT a requirement for a prescription to be considered valid under federal law?

  a. A DEA number for controlled substances

  b. The patient's date of birth

  c. The prescriber's signature

  d. The patient's name

62. The Drug Enforcement Administration (DEA) registration is required for:

  a. Patients receiving controlled substances

  b. Pharmacists dispensing controlled substances

  c. Prescribers prescribing controlled substances

  d. All of the above

63. Which federal law established the standards for tamper-evident packaging of over-the-counter (OTC) medications?

  a. FDCA

  b. DEA

  c. DQSA

  d. Federal Anti-Tampering Act

64. The FDA's REMS (Risk Evaluation and Mitigation Strategies) program is primarily aimed at:

a. Ensuring drug pricing transparency

b. Monitoring drug recalls

c. Managing the risks associated with certain medications

d. Regulating drug importation

65. Which federal law requires pharmacies to maintain records of controlled substance dispensing for at least two years?

a. CSA

b. FDCA

c. DSCSA

d. OBRA '90

66. Which federal agency oversees the National Drug Code (NDC) system?

a. FDA

b. DEA

c. CDC

d. FTC

67. What is the primary purpose of the Drug Supply Chain Security Act (DSCSA)?

    a. To regulate drug pricing

    b. To ensure the safety and traceability of the pharmaceutical supply chain

    c. To control drug importation

    d. To monitor drug recalls

68. Which federal law grants pharmacists the authority to administer vaccines to adults?

    a. FDCA

    b. ACA

    c. DSCSA

    d. VFC Program

69. What is the purpose of the Drug Efficacy Study Implementation (DESI) program?

    a. To regulate the importation of drugs

    b. To determine the safety and efficacy of older drugs

    c. To establish the scheduling of controlled substances

    d. To monitor drug recalls

70. Which federal law requires pharmacists to offer to counsel Medicaid patients regarding their prescriptions?

a. FDCA

b. HIPAA

c. ACA

d. OBRA '90

71. The Drug Price Competition and Patent Term Restoration Act (Hatch-Waxman Act) allows generic drug manufacturers to:

a. Extend the patent term of branded drugs

b. Bypass FDA approval for generic drugs

c. Challenge the patents of brand-name drugs

d. Set their own prices for generic drugs

72. Under the federal Combat Methamphetamine Epidemic Act, which of the following must be kept behind the pharmacy counter?

a. Syringes

b. Birth control pills

c. Pseudoephedrine-containing products

d. OTC pain relievers

73. Which federal agency is responsible for regulating the safety and labeling of cosmetics?

a. FDA

b. DEA

c. CDC

d. FTC

74. The federal law that established the Prescription Drug User Fee Act (PDUFA) allows the FDA to collect fees from:

a. Drug manufacturers to expedite the drug approval process

b. Patients to access prescription drug information

c. Pharmacies to maintain DEA registration

d. Medicaid beneficiaries

75. Which federal law created the Vaccine Adverse Event Reporting System (VAERS) to monitor the safety of vaccines?

a. CSA

b. FDCA

c. VAERS Act

d. ACA

76. Which federal agency enforces laws related to the labeling and advertising of tobacco products?

   a. FDA

   b. DEA

   c. CDC

   d. FTC

77. The Dietary Supplement Health and Education Act (DSHEA) allows dietary supplement manufacturers to make health claims on product labels without FDA approval.

   a. True

   b. False

78. Under federal law, who is responsible for ensuring that a prescription is valid and appropriate for the patient's condition?

   a. The patient

   b. The pharmacist

   c. The prescriber

   d. The insurance company

79. Which federal agency regulates the disposal of hazardous waste in healthcare settings, including pharmacies?

   a. FDA

   b. DEA

   c. CDC

   d. EPA

80. Which federal law established the National Vaccine Injury Compensation Program (VICP) to compensate individuals harmed by vaccines?

   a. FDCA

   b. ACA

   c. VICP Act

   d. DSCSA

81. The FDA Amendments Act (FDAAA) introduced a process called Risk Evaluation and Mitigation Strategies (REMS) to:

   a. Streamline the generic drug approval process

   b. Regulate the importation of drugs

   c. Ensure the safe use of certain medications

   d. Control drug pricing

82. What is the primary purpose of the Federal Combat Methamphetamine Epidemic Act (CMEA)?

a. To regulate the importation of methamphetamine

b. To combat the illegal production of methamphetamine

c. To provide treatment for individuals addicted to methamphetamine

d. To legalize the use of methamphetamine for medical purposes

83. Under the CMEA, which of the following products must be kept behind the pharmacy counter and sold only by a pharmacist or pharmacy technician?

a. Aspirin

b. Toothpaste

c. Pseudoephedrine-containing products

d. Over-the-counter vitamins

84. What is the maximum amount of pseudoephedrine-containing product that an individual can purchase in a single day under the CMEA without a prescription?

a. 3 grams

b. 7.5 grams

c. 9 grams

d. 12 grams

85. Which of the following is a requirement of the CMEA for retailers that sell pseudoephedrine-containing products?

  a. Retailers must maintain a logbook of pseudoephedrine sales.
  b. Retailers must provide counseling to customers purchasing these products.
  c. Retailers must refuse to sell any pseudoephedrine products.
  d. Retailers must offer discounts on pseudoephedrine products.

86. Which federal agency is responsible for enforcing the regulations outlined in the Combat Methamphetamine Epidemic Act (CMEA)?

  a. Food and Drug Administration (FDA)
  b. Drug Enforcement Administration (DEA)
  c. Centers for Disease Control and Prevention (CDC)
  d. Federal Trade Commission (FTC)

87. The CMEA requires retailers to verify the identity of purchasers of pseudoephedrine products by:

  a. Collecting a fingerprint
  b. Photocopying the purchaser's driver's license
  c. Scanning the purchaser's retina
  d. Checking a government-issued photo ID and recording the information

88. Which of the following is NOT a requirement for retailers under the CMEA?

    a. Retailers must limit sales to individuals 18 years of age or older.

    b. Retailers must maintain a logbook of sales.

    c. Retailers must provide counseling on the use of pseudoephedrine products.

    d. Retailers must report suspicious sales to the DEA.

89. The CMEA was enacted in response to:

    a. A surge in prescription drug abuse

    b. A rise in methamphetamine production and abuse

    c. A shortage of cold and allergy medications

    d. An increase in tobacco use

90. Which of the following individuals is exempt from the purchase restrictions on pseudoephedrine products under the CMEA?

    a. Anyone under the age of 21

    b. Individuals with a valid prescription

    c. Foreign tourists

    d. Retail employees

91. The CMEA imposes civil and criminal penalties for violations, including fines and imprisonment. Violations can result in penalties for:

    a. Retailers and purchasers

    b. Retailers only

    c. Purchasers only

    d. Manufacturers of pseudoephedrine products

92. What is the primary purpose of a Federal Pharmacy Patient Package Insert (PPI)?

    a. To provide dosage instructions to healthcare providers

    b. To contain pricing information for medications

    c. To offer comprehensive information to patients about their medications

    d. To track the expiration date of pharmaceutical products

93. Which federal agency mandates the inclusion of PPIs with certain prescription medications?

    a. Drug Enforcement Administration (DEA)

    b. Centers for Disease Control and Prevention (CDC)

    c. Food and Drug Administration (FDA)

    d. National Institutes of Health (NIH)

94. What information is typically included in a PPI?

a. Manufacturer's contact information only

b. Medication name and dosage form only

c. Dosage instructions, side effects, warnings, and other essential information

d. Prescription pricing and insurance details only

95. When should a pharmacist provide a PPI to a patient?

a. Only upon patient request

b. At the pharmacist's discretion

c. With every prescription medication, both new and refill orders

d. Only for controlled substances

96. Which of the following is NOT typically found in a PPI?

a. Dosage instructions

b. Manufacturer's contact information

c. Information on how to store the medication

d. Prescription pricing and insurance coverage details

97. What is the primary purpose of a Risk Evaluation and Mitigation Strategy (REMS) mandated by the FDA?

a. To promote the sales and marketing of pharmaceutical products

b. To facilitate the importation of specialty drugs

c. To ensure the safe use of certain medications with known risks

d. To streamline the approval process for generic drugs

98. Which federal agency is responsible for requiring REMS programs for specific medications?

a. Drug Enforcement Administration (DEA)

b. Centers for Disease Control and Prevention (CDC)

c. Food and Drug Administration (FDA)

d. National Institutes of Health (NIH)

99. What components are typically included in a REMS program?

a. Only medication pricing information

b. Patient education, prescriber certification, dispensing restrictions, and more

c. Manufacturer's contact information

d. Prescription drug importation details

100. When is a REMS program typically required for a medication?

a. Only for over-the-counter (OTC) medications

b. When the medication is first approved by the FDA

c. For all medications on the market

d. When the medication's patent expires

2. FEDERAL PHARMACY LAW ANSWERS PART-2

1. **Answer: C**

   Ensuring compliance with USP standards and performing quality checks.

   Explanation: Pharmacists are responsible for quality assurance in compounding, which includes adherence to USP standards and quality checks.

2. **Answer: A**

   To categorize drugs based on their potential for abuse and accepted medical use.

   Explanation: The classification helps in regulating their handling and distribution.

3. **Answer: C**

   DEA (Drug Enforcement Administration).

   Explanation: The DEA is responsible for regulating controlled substances, including scheduling.

4. **Answer: C**

   Methadone.

   Explanation: Methadone is an example of a Class II controlled substance used to treat opioid addiction.

5. **Answer: A**

   They have a high potential for abuse.

   Explanation: Class II controlled substances are known for their high potential for abuse and dependence.

6. **Answer: C**

Never, refills are not allowed.

Explanation: In general, Class II controlled substances do not permit refills.

7. **Answer: C**

The patient's name, prescriber's signature, and drug name.

Explanation: A valid prescription for a Class II controlled substance must include these essential elements.

8. **Answer: B**

Notify the DEA within one business day.

Explanation: Federal law requires pharmacies to report theft or loss of controlled substances to the DEA promptly.

9. **Answer: C**

Annually.

Explanation: Pharmacies are required to conduct an annual inventory of Class II controlled substances.

10. **Answer: B**

Explanation: Transfers are allowed once between pharmacies, under specific conditions and requirements.

11. **Answer: B**

The pharmacist must record the prescription in a central database.

Explanation: While some states have prescription monitoring programs, this is not a federal requirement for filling a Class II prescription.

12. **Answer: B**

Must be stored in a secure and retrievable manner.

Explanation: Prescription records for Class II controlled substances must be securely maintained for a specified period.

13. **Answer: C**

Based on a combination of their potential for abuse and medical use.

Explanation: Federal scheduling considers both the potential for abuse and accepted medical use.

14. **Answer: C**

To ensure the safe and secure handling of these substances.

Explanation: Federal regulations aim to prevent diversion and misuse of Class II controlled substances.

15. **Answer: B**

Medication's generic name.

Explanation: The label on dispensed prescription medications should include the medication's generic name, among other information.

16. **Answer: C**

Ensure the prescription is valid, including the prescriber's DEA number and patient information.

Explanation: Pharmacists must verify the legitimacy of Class II prescriptions.

17. **Answer: B**

They must be stored separately from other medications in a locked cabinet or safe.

Explanation: Class II controlled substances must be securely stored separately.

18. **Answer: D**

Schedule V.

Explanation: Schedule V substances have the lowest potential for abuse among controlled substances.

19. **Answer: C**

Both the transferring and receiving pharmacies must maintain records of the transfer.

Explanation: Documentation is required at both pharmacies involved in the transfer.

20. **Answer: B**

To prevent the diversion and abuse of these substances.

Explanation: The closed system aims to control and track Class II substances to prevent misuse.

21. **Answer: C**

Telepharmacy is allowed for Class II prescriptions under specific conditions.

Explanation: Telepharmacy may be used for Class II prescriptions as long as federal and state regulations are followed, including identity verification and record-keeping.

22. **Answer: C**

Providing false or misleading labeling or advertising for a drug.

Explanation: Misbranding occurs when a drug's labeling or advertising is inaccurate or deceptive

23. **Answer: C**

To educate patients about the drug's risks and benefits.

Explanation: Drug labeling is intended to inform patients and healthcare professionals about a drug's proper use and potential risks.

24. **Answer: C**

FDA (Food and Drug Administration).

Explanation: The FDA is responsible for enforcing regulations related to drug labeling and misbranding.

25. **Answer: D**

The drug is contaminated or unsafe for use.

Explanation: An adulterated drug is one that does not meet safety and quality standards.

26. **Answer: C**

Having a label that is difficult to read.

Explanation: While clear labeling is essential for patient safety, it does not typically result in a drug being considered adulterated.

27. **Answer: C**

To dispose of them immediately.

Explanation: Pharmacists should not dispense misbranded or adulterated drugs and should follow proper disposal procedures.

28. **Answer: C**

Drug facts labeling.

Explanation: OTC drugs must have drug facts labeling to provide consumers with information on proper use and potential risks.

29. **Answer: A**

The medication can only be dispensed with a prescription.

Explanation: The "Rx Only" label indicates that the medication requires a prescription.

30. **Answer: C**

To verify the accuracy of prescription labels and make corrections if necessary.

Explanation: Pharmacists play a crucial role in ensuring that prescription labels are accurate and compliant with federal regulations.

31. **Answer: C**

To create a database of all drugs in commercial distribution.

Explanation: The Drug Listing Act requires drug manufacturers and distributors to submit information about their products to the FDA's National Drug Code Directory. This helps maintain an accurate database of all drugs in commercial distribution.

32. **Answer: A**

FDA

Explanation: The Food and Drug Administration (FDA) is responsible for regulating prescription drugs' manufacturing and distribution.

33. **Answer: B**

HIPAA

Explanation: The Health Insurance Portability and Accountability Act (HIPAA) mandates patient privacy and confidentiality.

34. **Answer: A**

Schedule I

Explanation: Schedule I substances have the highest potential for abuse and are illegal for most purposes.

35. **Answer: B**

DEA

Explanation: The Drug Enforcement Administration (DEA) enforces controlled substance laws and regulations.

36. **Answer: B**

Generic drug approvals

Explanation: The Orange Book lists approved generic drugs and their therapeutic equivalence to brand-name drugs.

37. **Answer: C**

OBRA '90

Explanation: The Omnibus Budget Reconciliation Act of 1990 (OBRA '90) mandates counseling for Medicaid patients and drug utilization review.

38. **Answer: D**

DQSA

Explanation: The Drug Quality and Security Act (DQSA) regulates compounding by pharmacies and outsourcing facilities.

39. **Answer: D**

Drug traceability

Explanation: DSCSA focuses on ensuring the traceability and security of the pharmaceutical supply chain.

40. **Answer: A**

Kefauver-Harris Amendment

Explanation: The Kefauver-Harris Amendment gave the FDA authority to regulate drug marketing and promotion.

41. **Answer: C**

5 refills

Explanation: Federal law allows up to 5 refills for Schedule III controlled substances within 6 months.

42. **Answer: A**

HIPAA

Explanation: HIPAA established the NPI system and mandates its use for healthcare providers.

43. **Answer: B**

Drug safety and efficacy

Explanation: The FDCA primarily addresses drug safety and efficacy.

44. **Answer: D**

OBRA '90

Explanation: OBRA '90 mandates offering counseling on prescription drug use to all patients.

45. **Answer: A**

CSA

Explanation: The Controlled Substances Act (CSA) established the DEA.

46. **Answer: A**

FDA

Explanation: The FDA oversees and regulates clinical trials for new drugs.

47. **Answer: B**

Generic drug approval

Explanation: The Hatch-Waxman Act streamlines the approval process for generic drugs.

48. **Answer: A**

Registration of online pharmacies with the DEA

Explanation: The Ryan Haight Act requires online pharmacies to register with the DEA.

49. **Answer: A**

FDA

Explanation: The FDA regulates dietary supplements in the United States.

50. **Answer: C**

Product tampering of consumer goods

Explanation: The Federal Anti-Tampering Act addresses tampering with consumer products.

51. **Answer: A**

FDA

Explanation: The FDA regulates the labeling and advertising of OTC drugs.

52. **Answer: A**

Counterfeit drugs

Explanation: DQSA addresses concerns about counterfeit drugs and the safety of the drug supply.

53. **Answer: A**

CSA

Explanation: The Controlled Substances Act (CSA) laid the foundation for PDMPs.

54. **Answer: B**

7.5 grams

Explanation: Federal law limits non-prescription sales of pseudoephedrine-containing products to 7.5 grams per day.

55. **Answer: C**

FDA

Explanation: The FDA regulates the labeling and advertising of prescription drugs.

56. **Answer: B**

Regulates dietary supplement manufacturing

Explanation: DSHEA primarily regulates the manufacturing of dietary supplements.

57. **Answer: B**

BPCI Act

Explanation: The Biologics Price Competition and Innovation (BPCI) Act addresses biosimilar approval and regulation.

58. **Answer: B**

Orphan Drug Designation

Explanation: The Orphan Drug Act provides orphan drug designation to incentivize rare disease drug development.

59. **Answer: B**

Wholesaler

Explanation: Wholesalers are required to provide product tracing information under DSCSA.

60. **Answer: A**

HIPAA

Explanation: HIPAA allows patients to request access to their medical records.

61. **Answer: B**

The patient's date of birth

Explanation: The patient's date of birth is not required on a prescription.

62. **Answer: D**

All of the above

Explanation: DEA registration is required for patients, pharmacists, and prescribers involved with controlled substances.

63. **Answer: D**

Federal Anti-Tampering Act

Explanation: The Federal Anti-Tampering Act sets standards for tamper-evident packaging of OTC drugs.

64. **Answer: C**

Managing the risks associated with certain medications

Explanation: REMS is designed to manage the risks associated with specific drugs.

65. **Answer: A**

CSA

Explanation: The Controlled Substances Act (CSA) mandates record-keeping for controlled substances.

66. **Answer: A**

FDA

Explanation: The FDA oversees the NDC system, which identifies drugs.

67. **Answer: B**

To ensure the safety and traceability of the pharmaceutical supply chain

Explanation: DSCSA's primary purpose is to ensure the safety and traceability of the pharmaceutical supply chain.

68. **Answer: B**

ACA

Explanation: The Affordable Care Act (ACA) grants pharmacists the authority to administer vaccines to adults.

69. **Answer: B**

To determine the safety and efficacy of older drugs

Explanation: The DESI program evaluates the safety and efficacy of older drugs.

70. **Answer: D**

OBRA '90

Explanation: OBRA '90 mandates counseling for Medicaid patients.

71. **Answer: C**

Challenge the patents of brand-name drugs

Explanation: The Hatch-Waxman Act allows generic drug manufacturers to challenge the patents of brand-name drugs.

72. **Answer: C**

Pseudoephedrine-containing products

Explanation: The Combat Methamphetamine Epidemic Act requires pseudoephedrine products to be kept behind the pharmacy counter.

73. **Answer: A**

FDA

Explanation: The FDA regulates the safety and labeling of cosmetics.

74. **Answer: A**

Drug manufacturers to expedite the drug approval process

Explanation: PDUFA allows the FDA to collect fees from drug manufacturers to expedite drug approvals.

75. **Answer: C**

VAERS Act

Explanation: The VAERS Act established the Vaccine Adverse Event Reporting System.

76. **Answer: A**

FDA76.

Explanation: The FDA regulates the labeling and advertising of tobacco products.

77. **Answer: A**

True

Explanation: DSHEA allows dietary supplement manufacturers to make certain health claims without FDA preapproval.

78. **Answer: B**

The pharmacist

Explanation: Pharmacists are responsible for ensuring the validity and appropriateness of prescriptions.

79. **Answer: D**

EPA

Explanation: The Environmental Protection Agency (EPA) regulates the disposal of hazardous waste in healthcare settings.

80. **Answer: C**

VICP Act

Explanation: The VICP Act established the National Vaccine Injury Compensation Program.

81. **Answer: C**

Ensure the safe use of certain medications

Explanation: FDAAA introduced REMS to ensure the safe use of specific medications.

82. **Answer: B**

To combat the illegal production of methamphetamine

Explanation: The CMEA was enacted to combat the illegal production of methamphetamine by regulating the sale of pseudoephedrine-containing products, which are commonly used in the manufacturing of methamphetamine.

83. **Answer: C**

Pseudoephedrine-containing products

Explanation: The CMEA requires that products containing pseudoephedrine, such as cold and allergy medications, be kept behind the pharmacy counter and sold only by pharmacy staff.

84. **Answer: B**

7.5 grams

Explanation: The CMEA limits non-prescription sales of pseudoephedrine-containing products to 7.5 grams per day per individual.

85. **Answer: A**

Retailers must maintain a logbook of pseudoephedrine sales.

Explanation: The CMEA mandates that retailers selling pseudoephedrine-containing products must maintain a logbook to track sales, including purchaser information.

86. **Answer: B**

Drug Enforcement Administration (DEA)

Explanation: The DEA is responsible for enforcing the regulations related to pseudoephedrine-containing products under the CMEA.

87. **Answer: D**

Checking a government-issued photo ID and recording the information

Explanation: Retailers are required to check a government-issued photo ID, such as a driver's license, and record the purchaser's information when selling pseudoephedrine products.

88. **Answer: C**

Retailers must provide counseling on the use of pseudoephedrine products.

Explanation: While retailers are required to maintain a logbook and report suspicious sales, they are not required to provide counseling on the use of pseudoephedrine products under the CMEA.

89. **Answer: B**

A rise in methamphetamine production and abuse

Explanation: The CMEA was enacted to address the increase in methamphetamine production and abuse, particularly related to the diversion of pseudoephedrine-containing products.

90. **Answer: B**

Individuals with a valid prescription

Explanation: Individuals with a valid prescription for pseudoephedrine products are exempt from the purchase restrictions under the CMEA.

91. **Answer: A**

Retailers and purchasers

Explanation: The CMEA imposes penalties for both retailers and purchasers who violate its regulations, including fines and imprisonment.

92. **Answer: C**

To offer comprehensive information to patients about their medications

Explanation: The primary purpose of a PPI is to provide patients with essential information about their medications, including proper usage, side effects, and precautions.

93. **Answer: C**

Food and Drug Administration (FDA)

Explanation: The FDA mandates the inclusion of PPIs with certain prescription medications to ensure that patients receive critical information about their drugs.

94. **Answer: C**

Dosage instructions, side effects, warnings, and other essential information

Explanation: PPIs typically include dosage instructions, side effects, warnings, precautions, and other crucial information to help patients use their medications safely and effectively.

95. **Answer: C**

With every prescription medication, both new and refill orders

Explanation: Pharmacists are generally required to provide a PPI with every prescription medication, whether it's a new prescription or a refill, to ensure patients have access to essential drug information.

96. **Answer: D**

Prescription pricing and insurance coverage details

Explanation: PPIs typically do not contain information about prescription pricing or insurance coverage details. Their focus is on medication usage and safety information for patients.

97. **Answer: C**

To ensure the safe use of certain medications with known risks

Explanation: The primary purpose of a REMS is to mitigate known risks associated with certain medications and ensure their safe use by patients.

98. **Answer: C**

Food and Drug Administration (FDA)

Explanation: The FDA is responsible for mandating REMS programs for specific medications, particularly those with known safety concerns.

99. **Answer: B**

Patient education, prescriber certification, dispensing restrictions, and more

Explanation: REMS programs typically include multiple components, such as patient education, prescriber certification, dispensing restrictions, and more, to manage medication risks.

100. **Answer: B**

When the medication is first approved by the FDA

Explanation: REMS programs are usually required when a medication is initially approved by the FDA or when new safety concerns arise during its post-approval period.

3. FEDERAL PHARMACY LAW QUESTIONS PART-3

1. Which of the following is NOT a goal of a REMS program?

    a. To enhance patient access to medications

    b. To ensure the safe use of medications

    c. To minimize the risks associated with certain drug

    d. To prevent medication-related adverse events

2. Who has the primary responsibility for initiating a recall of a pharmaceutical product in the United States?

    a. The FDA

    b. The manufacturer or distributor

    c. The pharmacy

    d. The prescribing healthcare provider

3. Which federal agency oversees and enforces pharmaceutical recalls in the United States?

    a. Drug Enforcement Administration (DEA)

    b. Centers for Disease Control and Prevention (CDC)

    c. Food and Drug Administration (FDA)

    d. National Institutes of Health (NIH)

4. What is the primary reason for initiating a Class I pharmaceutical recall?

   a. To correct a minor labeling error

   b. To retrieve expired medications from the market

   c. To address a defect that could cause serious harm or death

   d. To reduce production costs

5. When a pharmacy receives notice of a drug recall, what is the most important initial action they should take?

   a. Continue dispensing the recalled product until it runs out of stock

   b. Quarantine the recalled product and stop dispensing it immediately

   c. Ignore the recall notice if the product is already in patients' hands

   d. Contact the prescribing healthcare provider for guidance

6. Which of the following is NOT a recommended step in handling a pharmaceutical recall at a pharmacy?

   a. Notify patients who have received the recalled product

   b. Document all actions related to the recall

   c. Wait for the FDA to provide instructions before taking any action

   d. Return the recalled product to the manufacturer or distributor

7. Which category of controlled substances includes medications with a moderate to low potential for physical and psychological dependence?

   a. Schedule I

   b. Schedule II

   c. Schedule III

   d. Schedule IV

8. Under federal law, which of the following healthcare providers can prescribe Schedule III and IV controlled substances?

   a. Physicians only

   b. Nurse practitioners and physician assistants

   c. Pharmacists

   d. Dentists only

9. What is the maximum allowable refill quantity for a Schedule III or IV controlled substance prescription under federal law?

   a. No refills allowed

   b. One refill

   c. Five refills within 6 months

   d. Unlimited refills

10. What is the typical duration of a Schedule III or IV controlled substance prescription, as allowed by federal law?

    a. 7 days

    b. 14 days

    c. 30 days

    d. 90 days

11. Which federal agency enforces the regulations surrounding Schedule III and IV controlled substances?

    a. Drug Enforcement Administration (DEA)

    b. Food and Drug Administration (FDA)

    c. Centers for Disease Control and Prevention (CDC)

    d. National Institutes of Health (NIH)

12. Which of the following is NOT a common Schedule IV controlled substance?

    a. Alprazolam (Xanax)

    b. Lorazepam (Ativan)

    c. Hydrocodone (Vicodin)

    d. Zolpidem (Ambien)

13. What is the primary factor that determines a controlled substance's placement into a specific schedule?

    a. Its potential for abuse

    b. Its cost

    c. Its chemical composition

    d. Its expiration date

14. Which schedule includes controlled substances with a high potential for abuse and no accepted medical use in the United States?

    a. Schedule I

    b. Schedule II

    c. Schedule III

    d. Schedule IV

15. What is the primary purpose of scheduling controlled substances into different categories (schedules)?

    a. To set maximum allowable prices for medications

    b. To facilitate international drug trade

    c. To regulate the manufacturing and distribution of controlled substances

    d. To increase the availability of medications to patients

16. Which of the following healthcare professionals can dispense Schedule III and IV controlled substances to patients?

    a. Pharmacists only

    b. Physicians only

    c. Dentists only

    d. Nurse practitioners, physician assistants, and pharmacists

17. According to federal law, how many times can a Schedule III to V prescription be transferred between pharmacies?

    a. Once

    b. Twice

    c. Three times

    d. An unlimited number of times

18. Which of the following healthcare professionals can initiate the transfer of a Schedule III to V prescription?

    a. Only the prescribing physician

    b. Pharmacists and pharmacy technicians

    c. Nurse practitioners and physician assistants

    d. All of the above

19. When transferring a Schedule III to V prescription, which piece of information is NOT typically required on the prescription transfer record?

   a. Name of the receiving pharmacy

   b. Date of the transfer

   c. Name of the pharmacist at the receiving pharmacy

   d. National Provider Identifier (NPI) of the prescribing healthcare provider

20. What is the maximum allowable time frame for completing the transfer of a Schedule III to V prescription, including the initial dispense?

   a. 7 days

   b. 14 days

   c. 30 days

   d. 90 days

21. What information must be communicated to the receiving pharmacy when transferring a Schedule III to V prescription?

   a. Only the prescription number

   b. Only the patient's name

   c. Prescrip21.tion number, patient's name, and the quantity dispensed

   d. Prescription number, patient's name, and the prescriber's name

22. In which schedule category does a medication with a moderate potential for abuse and accepted medical use fall?

    a. Schedule I

    b. Schedule II

    c. Schedule III

    d. Schedule IV

22. What is the primary federal law that governs the transfer of Schedule III to V prescriptions between pharmacies?

    a. The Controlled Substances Act (CSA)

    b. The Food, Drug, and Cosmetic Act (FDCA)

    c. The Affordable Care Act (ACA)

    d. The Poison Prevention Packaging Act (PPPA)

23. Which federal agency is responsible for enforcing the regulations related to controlled substances and prescription transfers?

    a. Drug Enforcement Administration (DEA)

    b. Centers for Medicare & Medicaid Services (CMS)

    c. Food and Drug Administration (FDA)

    d. National Institutes of Health (NIH)

25. What is the maximum allowable quantity of a Schedule III to V controlled substance that can be transferred between pharmacies?

   a. One day's supply

   b. A 72-hour supply

   c. A 30-day supply

   d. A 90-day supply

26. Under federal law, what is the minimum age requirement for a pharmacy technician to participate in the transfer of Schedule III to V prescriptions?

   a. 16 years old

   b. 18 years old

   c. 21 years old

   d. There is no minimum age requirement

27. Which federal program provides healthcare coverage primarily for individuals aged 65 and older, as well as some younger individuals with certain disabilities?

   a. Medicare

   b. Medicaid

   c. CHIP

   d. TRICARE

28. What is the primary federal agency responsible for administering the Medicare program?

   a. Centers for Disease Control and Prevention (CDC)

   b. Drug Enforcement Administration (DEA)

   c. Centers for Medicare & Medicaid Services (CMS)

   d. Food and Drug Administration (FDA)

29. Which part of Medicare covers prescription drug benefits for Medicare beneficiaries?

   a. Medicare Part A

   b. Medicare Part B

   c. Medicare Part C

   d. Medicare Part D

30. Medicaid is a joint federal and state program that provides healthcare coverage primarily for:

   a. Individuals aged 65 and older

   b. Low-income individuals and families

   c. Active-duty military personnel

   d. Veterans

31. Which federal agency oversees the Medicaid program and sets certain federal regulations and guidelines?

   a. Drug Enforcement Administration (DEA)

   b. Centers for Disease Control and Prevention (CDC)

   c. Centers for Medicare & Medicaid Services (CMS)

   d. Food and Drug Administration (FDA)

32. Which federal law expanded Medicaid eligibility to include more low-income adults in participating states?

   a. Social Security Act

   b. Affordable Care Act (ACA)

   c. Medicare Modernization Act (MMA)

   d. Medicaid Expansion Act

33. Pharmacies that participate in Medicare Part D must adhere to which set of regulations governing prescription drug coverage and claims processing?

   a. HIPAA regulations

   b. FDA regulations

   c. Medicare Part B regulations

   d. Medicare Part D regulations

34. Which of the following is NOT a factor considered when determining eligibility for Medicaid?

   a. Income

   b. Age

   c. Disability status

   d. Citizenship or immigration status

35. Which program provides healthcare coverage for low-income children in the United States?

   a. Medicare

   b. Medicaid

   c. CHIP

   d. TRICARE

36. What is the primary purpose of the Drug Utilization Review (DUR) program within Medicaid?

   a. To increase the cost of prescription medications

   b. To limit access to prescription drugs

   c. To ensure the safe and effective use of prescription medications

   d. To eliminate prescription drug coverage

37. Which federal agency is primarily responsible for regulating and enforcing laws related to controlled substances, including prescription medications with potential for abuse?

    a. Food and Drug Administration (FDA)

    b. Centers for Disease Control and Prevention (CDC)

    c. Drug Enforcement Administration (DEA)

    d. National Institutes of Health (NIH)

38. What is the primary mission of the DEA regarding controlled substances?

    a. To promote the pharmaceutical industry

    b. To reduce the availability of controlled substances

    c. To oversee clinical trials of new drugs

    d. To regulate the pricing of prescription medication

39. Which federal agency is responsible for approving new drugs for marketing in the United States and ensuring their safety and efficacy?

    a. Drug Enforcement Administration (DEA)

    b. Centers for Disease Control and Prevention (CDC)

    c. Food and Drug Administration (FDA)

    d. National Institutes of Health (NIH)

40. What is the primary purpose of the FDA's Center for Drug Evaluation and Research (CDER)?

   a. To regulate food products

   b. To evaluate and approve new drugs

   c. To enforce controlled substance laws

   d. To regulate the importation of medical devices

41. What is the FDA's role in the regulation of dietary supplements?

   a. The FDA does not regulate dietary supplements.

   b. The FDA strictly enforces regulations on dietary supplements.

   c. The FDA approves all dietary supplements before they can be sold.

   d. The FDA sets maximum pricing for dietary supplements.

42. Which federal agency is responsible for tracking and investigating outbreaks of foodborne illnesses and ensuring the safety of the food supply?

   a. Drug Enforcement Administration (DEA)

   b. Centers for Disease Control and Prevention (CDC)

   c. Food and Drug Administration (FDA)

   d. 42National Institutes of Health (NIH)

43. What is the primary function of the FDA's Center for Biologics Evaluation and Research (CBER)?

a. To regulate veterinary medications

b. To oversee the safety of vaccines and blood products

c. To enforce drug importation laws

d. To conduct clinical trials of new drugs

44. The Drug Enforcement Administration (DEA) assigns a unique registration number to:

a. Pharmaceutical manufacturers

b. Pharmacists

c. Patients

d. Prescribing healthcare providers

45. What is the primary purpose of the FDA's MedWatch program?

a. To regulate the importation of medical devices

b. To track adverse events and safety concerns related to medications and medical products

c. To conduct clinical trials of new drugs

d. To enforce food safety regulations

46. Which federal agency is responsible for regulating the labeling and advertising of tobacco products?

a. Drug Enforcement Administration (DEA)

b. Centers for Disease Control and Prevention (CDC)

c. Food and Drug Administration (FDA)

d. National Institutes of Health (NIH)

47. Which federal agency is primarily responsible for regulating medication development and marketing in the United States?

a. DEA

b. CDC

c. FDA

d. NIH

48. What does the acronym "DEA" stand for in the context of pharmacy law?

a. Drug Enforcement Administration

b. Drug Evaluation Agency

c. Drug Enforcement Act

d. Drug Expiration Agency

49. Which of the following is a key requirement for a drug to be classified as an over-the-counter (OTC) medication?

   a. Prescription-only status

   b. Available without a prescription

   c. Requires a physician's referral

   d. Available only to certain age groups

50. What does the Hatch-Waxman Act primarily relate to in the pharmaceutical industry?

   a. Drug pricing regulations

   b. Generic drug approval

   c. Drug patent extensions

   d. Drug manufacturing standards

51. What are REMS (Risk Evaluation and Mitigation Strategies) designed to address?

   a. Generic drug safety

   b. OTC medication labeling

   c. Medication advertising

   d. Risk management for certain medications

52. How does the FDA regulate the advertising and promotion of prescription drugs?

a. It has no authority over drug advertising.

b. It reviews and approves all drug advertisements.

c. It enforces regulations to ensure accurate and balanced drug promotion.

d. It relies solely on pharmaceutical companies to self-regulate advertising.

53. What is the primary purpose of the Orphan Drug Act?

a. To regulate drug importation

b. To encourage the development of medications for rare diseases

c. To regulate drug pricing

d. To promote generic drug competition

54. What do Good Manufacturing Practices (GMPs) primarily focus on in the pharmaceutical industry?

a. Drug pricing

b. Medication safety

c. Drug advertising

d. Drug importation

55. What are biosimilars in the context of medication regulation?

    a. Identical copies of brand-name drugs

    b. Generic versions of biologic drugs

    c. Specialty medications

    d. OTC medications

56. How does the Federal Anti-Tampering Act protect the integrity of over-the-counter medications?

    a. It regulates the pricing of OTC medications.

    b. It ensures the safety of OTC medication ingredients.

    c. It addresses tampering and contamination issues with OTC products.

    d. It mandates prescription-only status for OTC medications.

57. What role does the Federal Trade Commission (FTC) play in regulating medication advertising and marketing?

    a. It approves all medication advertisements.

    b. It enforces antitrust laws within the pharmaceutical industry.

    c. It oversees medication manufacturing standards.

    d. It reviews and approves medication labels.

58. What is the main focus of the Drug Supply Chain Security Act (DSCSA)?

a. Regulating drug prices

b. Ensuring medication accessibility

c. Enhancing medication safety and tracing

d. Promoting pharmaceutical advertising

59. Which federal agency primarily regulates the approval and oversight of biologic drugs in the United States?

a. Drug Enforcement Administration (DEA)

b. Federal Trade Commission (FTC)

c. Food and Drug Administration (FDA)

d. Centers for Disease Control and Prevention (CDC)

60. What distinguishes biologic drugs from traditional small-molecule drugs?

a. Biologics are always administered orally.

b. Biologics are synthesized through chemical processes.

c. Biologics are typically derived from living organisms.

d. Biologics have a longer shelf life.

61. What is the regulatory pathway for the approval of biosimilars in the United States?

a. Abbreviated New Drug Application (ANDA)

b. Biologics License Application (BLA)

c. New Drug Application (NDA)

d. Investigational New Drug Application (IND)

62. What role does the Purple Book play in the regulation of biologic drugs?

a. It provides information on drug pricing.

b. It lists approved biosimilar products.

c. It regulates drug advertising.

d. It addresses drug importation issues.

63. What does the Biologics Price Competition and Innovation Act (BPCIA) aim to achieve?

a. Regulating drug importation

b. Promoting the development of biosimilars

c. Ensuring drug accessibility

d. Regulating pharmaceutical advertising

64. What federal agency regulates and sets guidelines for the content and format of prescription drug labeling information for the patient?

    a. Drug Enforcement Administration (DEA)

    b. Federal Trade Commission (FTC)

    c. Food and Drug Administration (FDA)

    d. Centers for Disease Control and Prevention (CDC)

65. Which of the following is typically NOT included in the "Patient Information" section of prescription drug labeling?

    a. Dosage instructions

    b. Potential side effects

    c. Information on the drug's manufacturer

    d. How to store the medication

66. What is the purpose of the "Black Box Warning" in prescription drug labeling?

    a. To highlight the drug's brand name

    b. To emphasize the potential for severe or life-threatening side effects

    c. To indicate the drug's expiration date

    d. To list all possible drug interactions

67. Which of the following statements is true regarding the "Instructions for Use" section of prescription drug labeling?

   a. It provides information for healthcare professionals only.

   b. It offers guidance on how to administer the drug to patients.

   c. It includes pricing information for the medication.

   d. It is optional and not required by the FDA.

68. In the United States, what is the standard format for the "Drug Facts" label on over-the-counter (OTC) medications?

   a. The Physician Package Insert (PPI)

   b. The Medication Guide (MedGuide)

   c. The Prescription Drug Label (PDL)

   d. The Drug Facts panel

69. What is the primary distinction between pharmacy compounding and drug manufacturing?

   a. Compounding is performed by pharmacists, while manufacturing is done by pharmaceutical companies.

   b. Compounding is always done on a large scale, while manufacturing is typically small-scale.

   c. Compounding involves the creation of new drug formulations, while manufacturing produces existing drugs.

   d. Compounding is regulated by state pharmacy boards, while manufacturing is regulated by the FDA.

70. Which federal law specifically outlines the regulatory framework for pharmacy compounding?

a. Federal Food, Drug, and Cosmetic Act (FDCA)

b. Drug Quality and Security Act (DQSA)

c. Controlled Substances Act (CSA)

d. Dietary Supplement Health and Education Act (DSHEA)

71. What is the role of the United States Pharmacopeia (USP) in pharmacy compounding?

a. USP sets standards for the manufacturing of commercial drugs.

b. USP provides guidance for pharmacy compounding practices.

c. USP enforces regulations for controlled substances.

d. USP approves drug advertising.

72. Which of the following statements is true regarding the outsourcing of pharmacy compounding?

a. Outsourcing compounding facilities are subject to the same regulations as traditional pharmacies.

b. Outsourcing compounding facilities are not regulated by any federal agency.

c. Outsourcing compounding facilities are exempt from all compounding regulations.

d. Outsourcing compounding facilities are regulated solely by state pharmacy boards.

73. When does the FDA exercise its authority to regulate compounding pharmacies more like drug manufacturers?

a. When a compounding pharmacy operates in multiple states

b. When a compounding pharmacy uses bulk drug substances that are not on an FDA-approved list

c. When a compounding pharmacy provides compounded medications for individual patient prescriptions only

d. When a compounding pharmacy is a member of a professional pharmacy association

74. What is the "Orange Book" in the context of federal pharmacy law?

a. A reference book for prescription drug pricing information

b. A publication listing generic drug products and their equivalence to brand-name drugs

c. A regulatory document outlining drug manufacturing standards

d. A database of over-the-counter (OTC) medications

75. What does the term "AB rating" indicate in the Orange Book?

a. It signifies that a generic drug product is therapeutically equivalent to the brand-name drug.

b. It designates a brand-name drug's price.

c. It denotes a controlled substance classification.

d. It indicates the expiration date of a medication.

76. In what circumstances can a pharmacist substitute a brand-name drug with a generic drug without consulting the prescriber?

a. Only when the patient requests a generic

b. Never; pharmacists must always consult the prescriber before making substitutions

c. When the generic drug has an AB rating in the Orange Book

d. Only when the prescriber is unavailable for consultation

77. What is the role of the "Therapeutic Equivalence Codes" in the Orange Book?

a. They indicate the drug's shelf life.

b. They provide pricing information for generic drugs.

c. They specify the drug's dosage form.

d. They help healthcare professionals identify therapeutically equivalent drug products.

78. Which federal law governs the substitution of generic drugs for brand-name drugs by pharmacists?

a. Federal Food, Drug, and Cosmetic Act (FDCA)

b. Drug Price Competition and Patent Term Restoration Act (Hatch-Waxman Act)

c. Drug Enforcement Administration (DEA) regulations

d. Controlled Substances Act (CSA)

79. Which federal agency is primarily responsible for regulating and overseeing opioid treatment programs (OTPs) in the United States?

   a. Drug Enforcement Administration (DEA)

   b. Food and Drug Administration (FDA)

   c. Substance Abuse and Mental Health Services Administration (SAMHSA)

   d. Centers for Disease Control and Prevention (CDC)

80. What is the primary medication used in opioid treatment programs to help individuals with opioid use disorder?

   a. Methadone

   b. Oxycodone

   c. Fentanyl

   d. Hydrocodone

81. What are the main components of medication-assisted treatment (MAT) in opioid treatment programs?

   a. Medication, counseling, and psychosocial support

   b. Medication only

   c. Counseling and psychosocial support only

   d. Counseling only

82. What federal law allows qualified healthcare providers to prescribe buprenorphine for the treatment of opioid use disorder outside of traditional OTPs?

   a. Drug Addiction Treatment Act (DATA 2000)

   b. Controlled Substances Act (CSA)

   c. Drug Enforcement Administration (DEA) regulations

   d. Ryan Haight Online Pharmacy Consumer Protection Act

83. How are patients typically assessed for admission to an opioid treatment program (OTP)?

   a. Patients must pass a drug test.

   b. Patients are evaluated based on their insurance coverage.

   c. Patients are assessed for opioid use disorder through clinical evaluation.

   d. Patients must complete a counseling program.

84. What is the purpose of DEA Form 222 in federal pharmacy law?

   a. To register a pharmacy with the Drug Enforcement Administration (DEA)

   b. To report theft or loss of controlled substances

   c. To order Schedule II controlled substances for legitimate medical or research purposes

   d. To request authorization for the disposal of expired medications

85. Which of the following statements about DEA Form 222 is correct?

a. It can be used to order both Schedule II and Schedule III controlled substances.

b. It is an electronic form that can be submitted online.

c. It must be kept on file at the pharmacy for 30 days.

d. It requires the signature of both the supplier and the purchaser.

86. How many copies of DEA Form 222 are typically involved in the ordering process?

a. One copy

b. Two copies

c. Three copies

d. Four copies

87. In the event of a theft or loss of completed DEA Form 222, what should the pharmacy do?

a. Report it to the FDA

b. Report it to the DEA immediately

c. Keep it on file for future reference

d. Submit a copy to the state pharmacy board

88. Which federal agency enforces compliance with the regulations surrounding DEA Form 222?

a. Food and Drug Administration (FDA)

b. Drug Enforcement Administration (DEA)

c. Centers for Disease Control and Prevention (CDC)

d. Federal Trade Commission (FTC)

89. What is the primary purpose of a prescription monitoring program (PMP) in federal pharmacy law?

a. To regulate the pricing of prescription drugs

b. To monitor and track the prescribing and dispensing of controlled substances

c. To approve the marketing and advertising of prescription drugs

d. To establish guidelines for compounding pharmacies

90. Which healthcare professionals are typically required to report controlled substance prescriptions to a PMP?

a. Only pharmacists

b. Only prescribers (physicians, nurse practitioners, etc.)

c. Both pharmacists and prescribers

d. Only law enforcement agencies

91. How frequently are healthcare professionals usually required to report prescription data to a PMP?

a. Monthly

b. Annually

c. Quarterly

d. Daily

92. What is the main goal of using a PMP in the context of patient care?

a. To identify patients who are likely to misuse prescription medications

b. To restrict access to controlled substances for all patients

c. To replace the need for drug testing in pain management

d. To track the use of over-the-counter medications

93. In federal pharmacy law, who typically has access to the information stored in a PMP database?

a. The general public

b. Only pharmacists and prescribers

c. Law enforcement agencies

d. Only the DEA

94. What is the primary objective of the Omnibus Budget Reconciliation Act (OBRA) of 1990 concerning federal pharmacy law?

    a. To establish a national formulary for prescription medications

    b. To regulate the pricing of over-the-counter (OTC) medications

    c. To improve the quality of care in long-term care facilities through medication management

    d. To restrict the use of generic medications in favor of brand-name drugs

95. What key requirement did OBRA 1990 impose on pharmacists in the context of federal pharmacy law?

    a. Mandatory drug pricing disclosures to patients

    b. Mandatory counseling for Medicaid patients on new prescription medications

    c. Mandatory prescription compounding for Medicaid patients

    d. Mandatory pharmaceutical advertising for generic medications

96. Which federal agency oversees the implementation of OBRA 1990 provisions related to Medicaid and prescription drug coverage?

    a. Drug Enforcement Administration (DEA)

    b. Food and Drug Administration (FDA)

    c. Centers for Medicare & Medicaid Services (CMS)

    d. Substance Abuse and Mental Health Services Administration (SAMHSA)

97. What is the primary goal of the Drug Utilization Review (DUR) program mandated by OBRA 1990?

a. To promote the use of brand-name drugs over generic equivalents

b. To limit Medicaid beneficiaries' access to certain prescription medications

c. To prevent medication errors and ensure appropriate drug therapy

d. To reduce the number of pharmacies participating in Medicaid programs

98. How did OBRA 1990 impact the reimbursement of prescription medications for Medicaid beneficiaries?

a. It increased the cost-sharing requirements for beneficiaries.

b. It established a single, uniform reimbursement rate for all pharmacies.

c. It allowed for additional reimbursement to pharmacies for counseling services.

d. It eliminated prescription drug coverage for Medicaid beneficiaries.

99. What is the primary purpose of the Health Insurance Portability and Accountability Act (HIPAA) in the context of federal pharmacy law?

a. To regulate the pricing of prescription medications

b. To protect the privacy and security of patients' health information

c. To establish federal guidelines for pharmaceutical advertising

d. To standardize prescription drug labeling

100. Under HIPAA, what type of information is considered protected health information (PHI)?

a. Any information related to an individual's medical history

b. Any information related to an individual's insurance coverage

c. Any individually identifiable health information

d. Any information provided by a healthcare professional

3. FEDERAL PHARMACY LAW ANSWERS PART-3

1. **Answer: A**

   To enhance patient access to medications

   Explanation: While REMS programs aim to ensure the safe use of medications and minimize risks, their primary goal is not to enhance patient access. In some cases, REMS may include restrictions on access to ensure safe use.

2. **Answer: B**

   The manufacturer or distributor

   Explanation: The manufacturer or distributor of a pharmaceutical product has the primary responsibility for initiating a recall when safety concerns or product defects are identified.

3. **Answer: C**

   Food and Drug Administration (FDA)

   Explanation: The FDA is responsible for overseeing and enforcing pharmaceutical recalls to protect public health and safety.

4. **Answer: C**

   To address a defect that could cause serious harm or death

   Explanation: Class I recalls are initiated when there is a reasonable probability that the use of or exposure to a product will cause serious adverse health consequences or death.

5. **Answer: B**

Quarantine the recalled product and stop dispensing it immediately

Explanation: The most important initial action for a pharmacy is to quarantine the recalled product and stop dispensing it to prevent further distribution to patients.

6. **Answer: C**

Wait for the FDA to provide instructions before taking any action

Explanation: Pharmacies should not wait for FDA instructions but should take immediate action upon receiving a recall notice, including notifying patients, documenting actions, and returning the recalled product to the manufacturer or distributor when appropriate. Waiting for FDA instructions could delay necessary actions to protect patients' health.

7. **Answer: C**

Schedule III

Explanation: Schedule III controlled substances have a moderate to low potential for physical and psychological dependence compared to Schedule I and II substances.

8. **Answer: B**

Nurse practitioners and physician assistants

Explanation: Nurse practitioners and physician assistants, in addition to physicians, have the authority to prescribe Schedule III and IV controlled substances under federal law, subject to state regulations.

9. **Answer: C**

   Five refills within 6 months

   Explanation: Under federal law, Schedule III and IV controlled substance prescriptions can have up to five refills within a 6-month period.

10. **Answer: C**

    30 days

    Explanation: Federal law generally allows for a 30-day supply of Schedule III and IV controlled substances per prescription.

11. **Answer: A**

    Drug Enforcement Administration (DEA)

    Explanation: The DEA is responsible for enforcing regulations related to controlled substances, including Schedule III and IV drugs.

12. **Answer: C**

    Hydrocodone (Vicodin)

    Explanation: Hydrocodone is typically classified as a Schedule II controlled substance, not Schedule IV.

13. **Answer: A**

    Its potential for abuse

    Explanation: The potential for abuse i12s a primary factor in determining a controlled substance's schedule classification, with Schedule I having the highest potential for abuse and Schedule V having the lowest.

14. **Answer: A**

Schedule I

Explanation: Schedule I controlled substances have a high potential for abuse and no accepted medical use in the United States.

15. **Answer: C**

To regulate the manufacturing and distribution of controlled substances

Explanation: The primary purpose of scheduling controlled substances is to regulate their manufacturing, distribution, and use to prevent abuse and diversion.

16. **Answer: D**

Nurse practitioners, physician assistants, and pharmacists

Explanation: Nurse practitioners, physician assistants, and pharmacists, in addition to physicians, can dispense Schedule III and IV controlled substances to patients in accordance with federal and state regulations.

17. **Answer: B**

Twice

Explanation: Under federal law, a Schedule III to V prescription can be transferred between pharmacies only once. However, if it is not fully dispensed after the first transfer, it can be transferred one more time, totaling two transfers.

18. **Answer: D**

All of the above

Explanation: Under federal law, pharmacists, pharmacy technicians, nurse practitioners, physician assistants, and prescribing physicians can initiate the transfer of a Schedule III to V prescription, subject to state regulations.

19. **Answer: D**

National Provider Identifier (NPI) of the prescribing healthcare provider

Explanation: The NPI of the prescribing healthcare provider is not typically required on the prescription transfer record; instead, the name and DEA number of the prescriber are typically recorded.

20. **Answer: B**

14 days

Explanation: Federal law allows up to 14 days for completing the transfer of a Schedule III to V prescription, including the initial dispense by the receiving pharmacy.

21. **Answer: C**

Prescription number, patient's name, and the quantity dispensed

Explanation: When transferring a Schedule III to V prescription, federal law requires communication of the prescription number, patient's name, and the quantity dispensed to the receiving pharmacy.

22. **Answer: C**

Schedule III

Explanation: Medications with a moderate potential for abuse and accepted medical use are classified as Schedule III controlled substances.

23. **Answer: A**

The Controlled Substances Act (CSA)

Explanation: The transfer of Schedule III to V prescriptions between pharmacies is primarily governed by the Controlled Substances Act (CSA).

24. **Answer: A**

Drug Enforcement Administration (DEA)

Explanation: The DEA is responsible for enforcing the regulations related to controlled substances, including prescription transfers.

25. **Answer: C**

A 30-day supply

Explanation: The maximum allowable quantity of a Schedule III to V controlled substance that can be transferred between pharmacies is typically a 30-day supply.

26. **Answer: B**

18 years old

Explanation: Under federal law, pharmacy technicians involved in the transfer of Schedule III to V prescriptions must typically be at least 18 years old, although specific state requirements may vary.

27. **Answer: A**

Medicare

Explanation: Medicare is a federal program that primarily provides healthcare coverage for individuals aged 65 and older and some younger individuals with specific disabilities.

28. **Answer: C**

Centers for Medicare & Medicaid Services (CMS)

Explanation: CMS is the federal agency responsible for administering the Medicare program, including its prescription drug coverage, known as Medicare Part D.

29. **Answer: D**

Medicare Part D

Explanation: Medicare Part D is the part of Medicare that covers prescription drug benefits for Medicare beneficiaries.

30. **Answer: B**

Low-income individuals and families

Explanation: Medicaid is a joint federal and state program designed to provide healthcare coverage to low-income individuals and families.

31. **Answer: C**

Centers for Medicare & Medicaid Services (CMS)

Explanation: CMS is responsible for overseeing the Medicaid program at the federal level and establishing federal regulations and guidelines for the program.

32. **Answer: B**

Affordable Care Act (ACA)

Explanation: The Affordable Care Act (ACA) expanded Medicaid eligibility in participating states to include more low-income adults, increasing access to healthcare coverage.

33. **Answer: D**

Medicare Part D regulations

Explanation: Pharmacies that participate in Medicare Part D must adhere to the regulations specific to that program, including those related to prescription drug coverage and claims processing.

34. **Answer: B**

Age

Explanation: While age is a factor considered for Medicare eligibility, it is not a primary factor for Medicaid eligibility, which is primarily based on income, disability status, and citizenship or immigration status.

35. **Answer: C**

CHIP (Children's Health Insurance Program)

Explanation: CHIP is a federal program that provides healthcare coverage for low-income children in the United States, while Medicaid primarily serves low-income individuals and families.

36. **Answer: C**

To ensure the safe and effective use of prescription medications

Explanation: The Drug Utilization Review (DUR) program in Medicaid aims to ensure the safe and effective use of prescription medications by beneficiaries, rather than limiting access or increasing costs.

37. **Answer: C**

Drug Enforcement Administration (DEA)

Explanation: The DEA is the federal agency primarily responsible for regulating and enforcing laws related to controlled substances, ensuring their safe and legal use.

38. **Answer: B**

To reduce the availability of controlled substances

Explanation: The DEA's primary mission is to reduce the availability of controlled substances for illegal purposes while ensuring their availability for legitimate medical and scientific purposes.

39. **Answer: C**

Food and Drug Administration (FDA)

Explanation: The FDA is responsible for approving new drugs for marketing in the United States and overseeing their safety and efficacy throughout their lifecycle.

40. **Answer: B**

To evaluate and approve new drugs

Explanation: CDER within the FDA is responsible for evaluating and approving new drugs for marketing in the United States.

41. Answer: A

The FDA does not regulate dietary supplements.

Explanation: The FDA does not regulate dietary supplements in the same way it regulates prescription and over-the-counter drugs. Dietary supplements are regulated under the Dietary Supplement Health and Education Act (DSHEA).

42. Answer: B

Centers for Disease Control and Prevention (CDC)

Explanation: The CDC is responsible for tracking and investigating outbreaks of foodborne illnesses, while the FDA is primarily responsible for ensuring the safety of the food supply.

43. Answer: B

To oversee the safety of vaccines and blood products

Explanation: CBER within the FDA is responsible for regulating and ensuring the safety of vaccines, blood products, and related biologics.

44. Answer: B

Pharmacists

Explanation: The DEA assigns a unique registration number to pharmacists, allowing them to handle and dispense controlled substances.

45. Answer: B

To track adverse events and safety concerns related to medications and medical products

Explanation: The FDA's MedWatch program is designed to track and report adverse events and safety concerns related to medications and medical products.

46. Answer: C

Food and Drug Administration (FDA)

Explanation: The FDA is responsible for regulating the labeling and advertising of tobacco products under the Family Smoking Prevention and Tobacco Control Act.

47. Answer: C

FDA

Explanation: The Food and Drug Administration (FDA) is the primary federal agency responsible for regulating medication development, production, and marketing in the United States.

48. Answer: A

Drug Enforcement Administration

Explanation: The DEA, or Drug Enforcement Administration, plays a role in regulating controlled substances and enforcing drug-related laws.

49. Answer: B

Available without a prescription

Explanation: Over-the-counter (OTC) medications are available to consumers without a prescription, as opposed to prescription-only medications.

50. **Answer: B**

Generic drug approval

Explanation: The Hatch-Waxman Act is primarily related to the regulation and approval of generic drugs.

51. **Answer: D**

Risk management for certain medications

Explanation: REMS are strategies implemented by the FDA to manage and mitigate the risks associated with certain medications.

52. **Answer: C**

It enforces regulations to ensure accurate and balanced drug promotion.

Explanation: The FDA has authority over drug advertising and ensures that it is accurate and not misleading.

53. **Answer: B**

To encourage the development of medications for rare diseases

Explanation: The Orphan Drug Act provides incentives to pharmaceutical companies to develop medications for rare diseases.

54. **Answer: B**

Medication safety

GMPs ensure that pharmaceutical products are consistently produced and controlled to meet quality standards and safety requirements.

55. Answer: B

Generic versions of biologic drugs

Biosimilars are highly similar, but not identical, versions of biologic drugs.

56. Answer: C

It addresses tampering and contamination issues with OTC products.

Explanation: The Federal Anti-Tampering Act is designed to prevent tampering with consumer products, including OTC medications.

57. Answer: B

It enforces antitrust laws within the pharmaceutical industry.

Explanation: The FTC enforces competition and antitrust laws in various industries, including pharmaceuticals.

58. Answer: C

Enhancing medication safety and tracing

Explanation: The DSCSA aims to improve the security and traceability of the pharmaceutical supply chain.

59. Answer: C

Food and Drug Administration (FDA)

Explanation: The FDA is the primary federal agency responsible for regulating the approval, safety, and oversight of biologic drugs in the United States.

60. Answer: C

Biologics are typically derived from living organisms.

Explanation: Biologic drugs are typically large, complex molecules derived from living organisms or produced using biotechnology processes, while traditional small-molecule drugs are chemically synthesized.

61. Answer: B

Biologics License Application (BLA)

Explanation: Biosimilars are approved through the Biologics License Application (BLA) pathway, which is distinct from the pathway used for traditional small-molecule generic drugs (ANDA).

62. Answer: B

It lists approved biosimilar products.

Explanation: The Purple Book is a publication by the FDA that lists approved biologic products and their biosimilars, helping healthcare professionals and the public identify these products.

63. Answer: B

Promoting the development of biosimilars

Explanation: The BPCIA is a federal law that encourages the development and approval of biosimilars to increase competition and reduce the cost of biologic drugs.

64. Answer: C

Food and Drug Administration (FDA)

Explanation: The FDA is responsible for regulating and providing guidelines for prescription drug labeling information for the patient, ensuring it is accurate and informative.

65. Answer: C

Information on the drug's manufacturer

Explanation: The "Patient Information" section typically includes dosage instructions, potential side effects, and storage instructions, but it does not usually provide information on the drug's manufacturer.

66. Answer: B

To emphasize the potential for severe or life-threatening side effects

Explanation: A Black Box Warning is used to draw attention to serious or life-threatening risks associated with a medication.

67. Answer: B

It offers guidance on how to administer the drug to patients.

Explanation: The "Instructions for Use" section provides guidance on how patients should properly administer the medication, including any special instructions.

68. Answer: D

The Drug Facts panel

Explanation: The "Drug Facts" label is the standard format for presenting essential information on OTC medication packaging, required by the FDA to provide clear and concise information to consumers.

69. **Answer: A**

Compounding is performed by pharmacists, while manufacturing is done by pharmaceutical companies.

Explanation: The primary distinction is that compounding is the preparation of personalized medications by pharmacists or physicians for individual patients, while manufacturing is the large-scale production of commercial drug products by pharmaceutical companies.

70. **Answer: B**

Drug Quality and Security Act (DQSA)

Explanation: The Drug Quality and Security Act (DQSA) amended the FDCA to provide specific regulations and standards for pharmacy compounding.

71. **Answer: B**

USP provides guidance for pharmacy compounding practices.

Explanation: USP provides standards and guidance for the quality and safety of compounded medications, ensuring they meet specific requirements.

72. **Answer: A**

Outsourcing compounding facilities are subject to the same regulations as traditional pharmacies.

Explanation: Outsourcing compounding facilities must adhere to the same regulations and standards as traditional pharmacies to ensure the safety and quality of compounded medications.

73. Answer: B

When a compounding pharmacy uses bulk drug substances that are not on an FDA-approved list

Explanation: The FDA may exercise stricter regulatory oversight if a compounding pharmacy uses bulk drug substances that are not on an FDA-approved list or if other criteria are met, as outlined in the DQSA.

74. Answer: B

A publication listing generic drug products and their equivalence to brand-name drugs

Explanation: The Orange Book is a publication by the FDA that lists approved drug products, including generic drug products, and their therapeutic equivalence to brand-name drugs.

75. Answer: A

It signifies that a generic drug product is therapeutically equivalent to the brand-name drug.

Explanation: An AB rating in the Orange Book indicates that the generic drug product is considered therapeutically equivalent to the brand-name drug, allowing for substitution.

76. Answer: C

When the generic drug has an AB rating in the Orange Book

Explanation: Pharmacists can typically substitute a brand-name drug with a generic drug if the generic has an AB rating in the Orange Book, without the need for prescriber consultation.

77. Answer: D

They help healthcare professionals identify therapeutically equivalent drug products.

Explanation: Therapeutic Equivalence Codes in the Orange Book assist healthcare professionals in identifying drug products that are therapeutically equivalent to one another.

78. Answer: B

Drug Price Competition and Patent Term Restoration Act (Hatch-Waxman Act)

Explanation: The Hatch-Waxman Act establishes the legal framework for generic drug substitution by pharmacists in the United States.

79. Answer: C

Substance Abuse and Mental Health Services Administration (SAMHSA)

Explanation: SAMHSA is the federal agency responsible for regulating and overseeing OTPs to ensure the safe and effective treatment of opioid use disorder.

80. Answer: A

Methadone

Explanation: Methadone is a medication commonly used in opioid treatment programs to help individuals manage and overcome opioid addiction.

81. Answer: A

Medication, counseling, and psychosocial support

Explanation: MAT in opioid treatment programs typically includes medication, counseling, and psychosocial support to provide comprehensive treatment.

82. Answer: A

Drug Addiction Treatment Act (DATA 2000)

Explanation: DATA 2000 allows qualified healthcare providers to obtain a waiver to prescribe buprenorphine in office-based settings for opioid use disorder treatment.

83. Answer: C

Patients are assessed for opioid use disorder through clinical evaluation.

Explanation: Admission to an OTP usually involves a clinical evaluation to determine the presence and severity of opioid use disorder, which helps determine the appropriate treatment plan.

84. Answer: C

To order Schedule II controlled substances for legitimate medical or research purposes

Explanation: DEA Form 222 is used to order Schedule II controlled substances for legitimate medical or research purposes, serving as a record of the transaction.

85. Answer: D

It requires the signature of both the supplier and the purchaser.

Explanation: DEA Form 222 requires the signature of both the supplier (registrant) and the purchaser (pharmacy) to complete the order.

86. Answer: B

Two copies

Explanation: Typically, two copies of DEA Form 222 are involved in the ordering process: one is sent to the supplier, and the other is retained by the purchaser.

87. Answer: B

Report it to the DEA immediately

Explanation: In the event of a theft or loss of a completed DEA Form 222, the pharmacy should report it to the DEA immediately to prevent unauthorized orders.

88. Answer: B

Drug Enforcement Administration (DEA)

Explanation: The DEA is responsible for enforcing compliance with the regulations surrounding DEA Form 222 and controlled substance ordering.

89. Answer: B

To monitor and track the prescribing and dispensing of controlled substances

Explanation: The primary purpose of a PMP is to monitor and track the prescribing and dispensing of controlled substances to help prevent misuse and diversion.

90. Answer: C

Both pharmacists and prescribers

Explanation: Both pharmacists and prescribers are typically required to report controlled substance prescriptions to a PMP to ensure comprehensive tracking.

91. Answer: D

Daily

Explanation: In many jurisdictions, healthcare professionals are required to report prescription data to a PMP on a daily basis to provide up-to-date information.

92. Answer: A

To identify patients who are likely to misuse prescription medications

Explanation: One of the primary goals of a PMP is to identify patients who may be at risk of misusing or abusing prescription medications so that appropriate interventions can be implemented.

93. Answer: C

Only pharmacists and prescribers

Explanation: Generally, only pharmacists and prescribers with a legitimate need to access PMP data are granted access to the information for patient care purposes, not the general public.

94. Answer: C

To improve the quality of care in long-term care facilities through medication management

Explanation: OBRA 1990 included provisions to enhance the quality of care for residents in long-term care facilities, emphasizing medication management and the role of pharmacists.

95. Answer: B

Mandatory counseling for Medicaid patients on new prescription medications

Explanation: OBRA 1990 required pharmacists to offer counseling to Medicaid patients receiving new prescription medications to ensure they understood proper medication use.

96. Answer: C

Centers for Medicare & Medicaid Services (CMS)

Explanation: CMS oversees the implementation of OBRA 1990 provisions related to Medicaid and prescription drug coverage.

97. Answer: C

To prevent medication errors and ensure appropriate drug therapy

Explanation: The DUR program required states to establish procedures for prospective and retrospective drug use reviews to prevent medication errors and ensure appropriate drug therapy.

98. Answer: C

It allowed for additional reimbursement to pharmacies for counseling services. Explanation: OBRA 1990 provided for additional reimbursement to pharmacies for the provision of counseling services to Medicaid beneficiaries, incentivizing pharmacists to offer counseling as required.

99. Answer: B

To protect the privacy and security of patients' health information

Explanation: HIPAA's primary purpose is to safeguard the privacy and security of patients' protected health information (PHI), including their medical and prescription records.

100. Answer: C

Any individually identifiable health information

Explanation: PHI includes any individually identifiable health information, such as medical records, prescriptions, and billing information.

4. FEDERAL PHARMACY LAW QUESTIONS PART-4

1. Which healthcare entity or provider is considered a covered entity under HIPAA and is subject to its privacy and security regulations?

   a. Pharmacies only

   b. Health insurance companies only

   c. Healthcare providers, health plans, and healthcare clearinghouses

   d. Patients and their families

2. What is the minimum standard required by HIPAA for the protection of electronic protected health information (ePHI)?

   a. Encryption is optional for ePHI.

   b. Access to ePHI must be completely unrestricted.

   c. Reasonable safeguards must be in place to protect ePHI.

   d. ePHI cannot be stored electronically.

3. What is the role of the Health and Human Services (HHS) Office for Civil Rights (OCR) in enforcing HIPAA regulations?

   a. HHS OCR provides technical support for covered entities.

   b. HHS OCR investigates and enforces compliance with HIPAA rules.

   c. HHS OCR manages prescription drug pricing.

   d. HHS OCR is responsible for advertising approvals.

4. What is the primary purpose of federal antitrust laws in the context of pharmacy and healthcare?

   a. To regulate the pricing of prescription medications

   b. To promote competition and prevent anti-competitive practices

   c. To establish federal guidelines for pharmaceutical advertising

   d. To regulate the importation of prescription drugs

5. Which federal antitrust law is primarily concerned with preventing monopolistic practices and promoting fair competition in commerce?

   a. Sherman Antitrust Act

   b. Federal Trade Commission Act

   c. Food, Drug, and Cosmetic Act

   d. Drug Price Competition and Patent Term Restoration Act (Hatch-Waxman Act)

6. Which of the following actions could be considered a violation of federal antitrust laws in the pharmacy industry?

   a. A group of pharmacies negotiating collectively with drug manufacturers for better pricing

   b. A pharmacy chain offering loyalty rewards to customers

   c. An independent pharmacy competing aggressively on pricing

   d. A pharmacy refusing to stock a certain brand of medication

7. How do federal antitrust laws relate to pharmacy mergers and acquisitions?

   a. Federal antitrust laws encourage pharmacy mergers to reduce competition.

   b. Federal antitrust laws prohibit pharmacy mergers and acquisitions.

   c. Federal antitrust laws may scrutinize pharmacy mergers that could harm competition.

   d. Federal antitrust laws do not apply to pharmacy mergers.

8. What federal agency is responsible for enforcing federal antitrust laws in the United States?

   a. Food and Drug Administration (FDA)

   b. Drug Enforcement Administration (DEA)

   c. Federal Trade Commission (FTC)

   d. Centers for Medicare & Medicaid Services (CMS)

9. What is a malpractice action in the context of federal pharmacy law?

   a. A lawsuit against a pharmacy for dispensing generic drugs

   b. A legal claim against a healthcare provider, including pharmacists, for negligence or professional misconduct

   c. A federal law regulating drug pricing

   d. A legal action taken by a patient to obtain a prescription refill

10. What is a key element that a plaintiff must establish in a malpractice action against a pharmacist?

    a. The pharmacist's educational background

    b. The pharmacist's licensure status

    c. The pharmacist's intent to harm the patient

    d. The pharmacist's breach of the standard of care

11. Which federal law governs the liability of pharmacists and other healthcare providers in malpractice actions?

    a. Controlled Substances Act (CSA)

    b. Drug Price Competition and Patent Term Restoration Act (Hatch-Waxman Act)

    c. Health Insurance Portability and Accountability Act (HIPAA)

    d. State law, as federal law generally does not govern malpractice actions

12. In a malpractice action, what is the role of expert witnesses?

    a. To provide character references for the healthcare provider

    b. To testify about the standard of care and whether it was breached

    c. To act as legal advisors to the plaintiff

    d. To determine the damages awarded to the plaintiff

13. Which of the following is a potential outcome of a successful malpractice action?

    a. Criminal charges filed against the pharmacist

    b. Revocation of the pharmacist's license

    c. Monetary damages awarded to the plaintiff

    d. Federal prosecution under the Drug Enforcement Administration (DEA)

14. What is the primary purpose of repository or take-back programs in federal pharmacy law?

    a. To provide free medications to low-income individuals

    b. To regulate the pricing of prescription medications

    c. To ensure the proper disposal of unused or expired medications

    d. To facilitate the importation of prescription drugs

15. Which federal agency provides guidance and regulations related to the establishment and operation of medication repository or take-back programs?

    a. Drug Enforcement Administration (DEA)

    b. Food and Drug Administration (FDA)

    c. Centers for Medicare & Medicaid Services (CMS)

    d. Substance Abuse and Mental Health Services Administration (SAMHSA)

16. What types of medications are typically accepted in repository or take-back programs?

    a. All prescription and over-the-counter medications

    b. Only controlled substances

    c. Only expired medications

    d. Only brand-name medications

17. What is the goal of the Secure and Responsible Drug Disposal Act of 2010 in federal pharmacy law?

    a. To promote the sale of expired medications

    b. To establish medication recycling programs

    c. To facilitate the return of controlled substances to pharmacies

    d. To provide funding for prescription assistance programs

18. In the context of repository or take-back programs, what does "stewardship" refer to?

    a. The process of selling unused medications to pharmacies

    b. The responsibility of pharmacies to provide free medications to patients

    c. The management and oversight of medication disposal programs

    d. The process of importing medications from other countries

19. What is drug product liability in the context of federal pharmacy law?

a. The legal responsibility of pharmacies to provide prescription medications to patients

b. The liability of manufacturers, distributors, and sellers of drugs for harm caused by defective or dangerous products

c. The requirement for pharmacies to maintain a liability insurance policy

d. The legal protection afforded to pharmacists against malpractice claims

20. Which legal theory is commonly used in drug product liability cases when a plaintiff alleges that a drug manufacturer failed to warn about known risks associated with the medication?

a. Strict liability

b. Res ipsa loquitur

c. Negligence

d. Intentional tort

21. In a drug product liability case, what does "failure to warn" refer to?

a. The pharmacy's failure to provide medication counseling to the patient

b. The manufacturer's failure to warn healthcare providers about the drug's potential side effects

c. The manufacturer's failure to adequately warn consumers and healthcare providers about known risks and side effects of a drug

d. The distributor's failure to maintain proper storage conditions for the drug

22. Which federal agency regulates drug product labeling and requires manufacturers to include specific information about a drug's risks and benefits?

    a. Drug Enforcement Administration (DEA)

    b. Food and Drug Administration (FDA)

    c. Centers for Medicare & Medicaid Services (CMS)

    d. Federal Trade Commission (FTC)

23. What is the primary goal of drug product liability laws and regulations in federal pharmacy law?

    a. To protect pharmacies from liability claims

    b. To encourage the sale of prescription medications

    c. To ensure that manufacturers and distributors of drugs produce safe and effective products

    d. To provide free legal services to patients harmed by medications

24. What is the primary purpose of risk management strategies in federal pharmacy law?

    a. To increase the cost of prescription medications

    b. To limit patient access to prescription medications

    c. To identify, mitigate, and prevent risks associated with pharmaceutical products and services

    d. To regulate the marketing of over-the-counter (OTC) medications

25. Which federal agency plays a central role in the development and oversight of risk evaluation and mitigation strategies (REMS) for certain medications?

    a. Drug Enforcement Administration (DEA)

    b. Food and Drug Administration (FDA)

    c. Centers for Medicare & Medicaid Services (CMS)

    d. Substance Abuse and Mental Health Services Administration (SAMHSA)

26. What is the primary goal of a risk evaluation and mitigation strategy (REMS) program for a medication?

    a. To increase the medication's availability and accessibility

    b. To encourage healthcare providers to prescribe the medication

    c. To ensure the safe use of a medication with known risks

    d. To promote the medication's off-label use

27. In the context of federal pharmacy law, what is a Medication Guide, and when is it typically required?

    a. A prescription label attached to every medication container

    b. A patient education document providing essential information about certain prescription medications, typically required when the FDA determines that patient adherence is crucial

    c. A warning letter from the FDA to healthcare providers about the risks of a specific medication

    d. A document provided to pharmacists during medication recalls

28. Which of the following is an example of a risk management strategy implemented by pharmacies to prevent medication errors?

    a. Offering discounts on prescription medications

    b. Providing medication therapy management (MTM) services

    c. Promoting the use of brand-name medications over generics

    d. Stocking expired medications on the shelves

29. What is the primary purpose of record-keeping requirements in federal pharmacy law?

    a. To increase the cost of healthcare services

    b. To maintain a historical account of all pharmacy transactions

    c. To regulate the pricing of prescription medications

    d. To protect patient health and safety

30. Which federal agency sets and enforces record-keeping requirements for pharmacies in the United States?

    a. Drug Enforcement Administration (DEA)

    b. Food and Drug Administration (FDA)

    c. Centers for Medicare & Medicaid Services (CMS)

    d. Substance Abuse and Mental Health Services Administration (SAMHSA)

31. How long are most pharmacies required to maintain prescription records for controlled substances under federal law?

    a. 1 year

    b. 3 years

    c. 5 years

    d. 10 years

32. In addition to prescription records, what other types of records are typically required to be maintained by pharmacies under federal pharmacy law?

    a. Employee payroll records

    b. Customer purchase histories

    c. Inventory and drug order records

    d. Marketing and advertising materials

33. What is the main consequence for a pharmacy that fails to comply with federal record-keeping requirements?

    a. Immediate suspension of the pharmacy's license

    b. Criminal prosecution of the pharmacy owner

    c. Monetary fines and penalties

    d. Loss of DEA registration and ability to handle controlled substances

34. What federal agency is primarily responsible for the classification and regulation of controlled substances in the United States?

    a. Drug Enforcement Administration (DEA)

    b. Food and Drug Administration (FDA)

    c. Centers for Disease Control and Prevention (CDC)

    d. Department of Health and Human Services (HHS)

35. Which schedule of controlled substances includes drugs with the highest potential for abuse and no accepted medical use in the United States?

    a. Schedule I

    b. Schedule II

    c. Schedule III

    d. Schedule IV

36. Which schedule of controlled substances includes medications with a lower potential for abuse and accepted medical use, but still requires strict record-keeping and prescription requirements?

    a. Schedule I

    b. Schedule II

    c. Schedule III

    d. Schedule IV

37. Which of the following factors is NOT considered when classifying a substance into a particular schedule under federal pharmacy law?

    a. The substance's potential for abuse

    b. The substance's chemical structure

    c. The substance's medical use and accepted safety for use under medical supervision

    d. The substance's market demand and pricing

38. What is the primary purpose of classifying drugs into schedules under the Controlled Substances Act (CSA)?

    a. To ensure that all medications are available without restrictions

    b. To create a standardized pricing system for prescription drugs

    c. To regulate the manufacture, distribution, and dispensing of controlled substances based on their potential for abuse

    d. To limit the availability of generic medications

39. Which schedule typically includes medications that are available without a prescription (over-the-counter)?

    a. Schedule I

    b. Schedule II

    c. Schedule III

    d. Schedule V

40. Which schedule includes medications like codeine-containing cough syrups when used in combination with other non-narcotic ingredients?

    a. Schedule I

    b. Schedule II

    c. Schedule III

    d. Schedule V

41. Which schedule of controlled substances includes anabolic steroids used for performance enhancement?

    a. Schedule I

    b. Schedule II

    c. Schedule III

    d. Schedule IV

42. Which federal agency has the authority to reschedule or de-schedule controlled substances under the Controlled Substances Act (CSA)?

    a. Drug Enforcement Administration (DEA)

    b. Food and Drug Administration (FDA)

    c. Centers for Medicare & Medicaid Services (CMS)

    d. National Institutes of Health (NIH)

43. In which schedule are medications like Xanax (alprazolam) and Valium (diazepam) classified?

   a. Schedule I

   b. Schedule II

   c. Schedule III

   d. Schedule IV

44. Which schedule includes medications like Vicodin (hydrocodone/acetaminophen) and OxyContin (oxycodone)?

   a. Schedule I

   b. Schedule II

   c. Schedule III

   d. Schedule IV

45. What is the primary responsibility of pharmacies when handling controlled substances under federal pharmacy law?

   a. To promote the use of controlled substances

   b. To limit the availability of controlled substances to healthcare providers only

   c. To maintain accurate records of controlled substance transactions

   d. To conduct clinical trials on controlled substances

46. Under federal pharmacy law, who is typically allowed to prescribe Schedule II controlled substances?

    a. Only medical doctors (MDs)

    b. Only dentists

    c. Medical doctors (MDs), dentists, and nurse practitioners (NPs)

    d. Only pharmacists

47. What is the primary requirement for transferring a Schedule III or IV prescription from one pharmacy to another under federal pharmacy law?

    a. The receiving pharmacy must notify the DEA

    b. The patient must provide written consent for the transfer

    c. The transfer must occur within 7 days of the original prescription date

    d. Only electronic transfers are allowed

48. Which schedule of controlled substances includes medications with a moderate potential for abuse and accepted medical use, often with limited refills?

    a. Schedule I

    b. Schedule II

    c. Schedule III

    d. Schedule IV

49. Which federal law established the scheduling system for controlled substances in the United States?

    a. The Food, Drug, and Cosmetic Act (FDCA)

    b. The Drug Price Competition and Patent Term Restoration Act (Hatch-Waxman Act)

    c. The Controlled Substances Act (CSA)

    d. The Prescription Drug Marketing Act (PDMA)

50. Which schedule includes medications like Tylenol with codeine?

    a. Schedule I

    b. Schedule II

    c. Schedule III

    d. Schedule IV

51. What is the primary difference between Schedule II and Schedule III controlled substances regarding prescription refills?

    a. Schedule II medications cannot be refilled, while Schedule III medications can have limited refills

    b. Schedule II medications can have unlimited refills, while Schedule III medications cannot be refilled

    c. Both Schedule II and Schedule III medications cannot be refilled

    d. Both Schedule II and Schedule III medications can have unlimited refills

52. What federal pharmacy law provision requires pharmacies to maintain separate records for controlled substances and non-controlled substances?

    a. The Controlled Substances Act (CSA)

    b. The Food, Drug, and Cosmetic Act (FDCA)

    c. The Drug Price Competition and Patent Term Restoration Act (Hatch-Waxman Act)

    d. The Prescription Drug Marketing Act (PDMA)

53. In the context of controlled substance scheduling, what does "DEA registration" refer to?

    a. The process of patients registering to receive controlled substances

    b. The unique registration number issued to healthcare providers and pharmacies by the DEA

    c. The requirement for pharmacies to register with the FDA

    d. The process of scheduling controlled substances

54. Under federal pharmacy law, which schedule of controlled substances can be transferred between pharmacies without restrictions, including Schedule II?

    a. Schedule I

    b. Schedule II

    c. Schedule III

    d. Schedule IV

55. What is the primary reason for allowing the transfer of Schedule III, IV, and V controlled substance prescriptions between pharmacies?

    a. To make it easier for patients to obtain controlled substances

    b. To reduce the workload of pharmacies

    c. To ensure that patients have access to needed medications

    d. To eliminate the need for record-keeping

56. How many times can a Schedule III, IV, or V controlled substance prescription be transferred between pharmacies?

    a. Only once

    b. Up to three times

    c. As many times as needed

    d. No transfers are allowed

57. When transferring a Schedule III, IV, or V controlled substance prescription, what information must be documented on the transferring pharmacy's records?

    a. The patient's name, address, and phone number

    b. The pharmacist's signature

    c. The date of transfer and the receiving pharmacy's name and address

    d. The medication's lot number

58. What is the primary limitation on transferring a Schedule II controlled substance prescription between pharmacies?

    a. Transfers are never allowed for Schedule II prescriptions.

    b. It can only be transferred once.

    c. It can be transferred up to five times.

    d. It can be transferred only to pharmacies within the same state.

59. When a Schedule III, IV, or V controlled substance prescription is transferred, who is responsible for ensuring that the patient does not receive more medication than prescribed?

    a. The transferring pharmacist

    b. The receiving pharmacist

    c. The patient's physician

    d. The pharmacy technician

60. Under federal pharmacy law, when can a pharmacy receive a faxed prescription for a Schedule II controlled substance?

    a. Only when the patient is in a long-term care facility

    b. Only when the pharmacy has a special waiver

    c. Never; faxed prescriptions for Schedule II substances are not allowed

    d. Always, as long as the fax includes the prescribing physician's DEA number

61. What additional requirement must be met when a faxed prescription for a Schedule II controlled substance is received by a pharmacy?

    a. The prescription must be handwritten by the prescribing physician.

    b. The prescribing physician must confirm the prescription with a follow-up phone call.

    c. The pharmacy must obtain the original hard copy of the prescription within 7 days.

    d. The pharmacy must notify the DEA immediately.

62. In which circumstances can a pharmacy receive a faxed prescription for a Schedule III, IV, or V controlled substance?

    a. Only when the pharmacy has a special waiver

    b. Only when the prescribing physician is out of state

    c. When the patient is in a long-term care facility or for compound prescriptions

    d. Never; faxed prescriptions for these substances are not allowed

63. What information must be included on a faxed prescription for a controlled substance to be valid under federal law?

    a. The patient's name and address

    b. The pharmacy's DEA registration number

    c. The prescribing physician's signature

    d. The pharmacy's contact information

4. FEDERAL PHARMACY LAW ANSWERS PART-4

1. **Answer: C**

   Healthcare providers, health plans, and healthcare clearinghouses

   Explanation: Covered entities under HIPAA include healthcare providers, health plans, and healthcare clearinghouses, which may encompass pharmacies, hospitals, insurance companies, and more.

2. **Answer: C**

   Reasonable safeguards must be in place to protect ePHI.

   Explanation: HIPAA requires covered entities to implement reasonable safeguards to protect ePHI, including encryption, access controls, and audit logs.

3. **Answer: B**

   HHS OCR investigates and enforces compliance with HIPAA rules.

   Explanation: The HHS OCR is responsible for investigating and enforcing compliance with HIPAA rules, ensuring that covered entities protect patients' privacy and security.

4. **Answer: B**

   To promote competition and prevent anti-competitive practices

   Explanation: Federal antitrust laws are designed to promote competition, prevent monopolies, and prohibit anti-competitive practices that could harm consumers or competition in the marketplace.

5. **Answer: A**

Sherman Antitrust Act

Explanation: The Sherman Antitrust Act is the primary federal antitrust law aimed at preventing monopolies and promoting fair competition in commerce.

6. **Answer: A**

A group of pharmacies negotiating collectively with drug manufacturers for better pricing

Explanation: Collective negotiation by a group of pharmacies may raise concerns under federal antitrust laws if it reduces competition in the marketplace.

7. **Answer: C**

Federal antitrust laws may scrutinize pharmacy mergers that could harm competition.

Explanation: Federal antitrust laws may review and scrutinize pharmacy mergers and acquisitions if there are concerns that they could reduce competition in the pharmacy market.

8. **Answer: C**

Federal Trade Commission (FTC)

Explanation: The Federal Trade Commission (FTC) is responsible for enforcing federal antitrust laws in the United States, including those related to pharmacy and healthcare.

9. **Answer: B**

A legal claim against a healthcare provider, including pharmacists, for negligence or professional misconduct

Explanation: A malpractice action is a legal claim brought against healthcare providers, including pharmacists, for negligence or professional misconduct in providing patient care.

10. **Answer: D**

The pharmacist's breach of the standard of care

Explanation: To succeed in a malpractice action, a plaintiff must typically establish that the pharmacist breached the standard of care, which means failing to provide the level of care that a reasonably prudent pharmacist would provide in similar circumstances.

11. **Answer: D**

State law, as federal law generally does not govern malpractice actions

Explanation: Malpractice actions are primarily governed by state law, and the specifics can vary from one state to another. Federal law typically does not regulate the liability of healthcare providers in malpractice actions.

12. **Answer: C**

To testify about the standard of care and whether it was breached

Explanation: Expert witnesses play a crucial role in malpractice actions by providing testimony about the standard of care and whether the defendant healthcare provider breached it.

13. **Answer: C**

Monetary damages awarded to the plaintiff

Explanation: In a successful malpractice action, the plaintiff may be awarded monetary damages as compensation for harm or injuries resulting from the negligence or misconduct of the healthcare provider.

14. **Answer: C**

To ensure the proper disposal of unused or expired medications

Explanation: Repository or take-back programs are designed to collect and dispose of unused or expired medications safely, reducing the risk of diversion and environmental contamination.

15. **Answer: B**

Food and Drug Administration (FDA)

Explanation: The FDA provides guidance and regulations related to the establishment and operation of medication repository or take-back programs.

16. **Answer: A**

All prescription and over-the-counter medications

Explanation: Most repository or take-back programs accept all prescription and over-the-counter medications to ensure comprehensive disposal options for the public.

17. Answer: C

To facilitate the return of controlled substances to pharmacies

Explanation: The Secure and Responsible Drug Disposal Act of 2010 amended the Controlled Substances Act to allow for the return of controlled substances to authorized pharmacies for disposal.

18. Answer: C

The management and oversight of medication disposal programs

Explanation: In the context of repository or take-back programs, "stewardship" refers to the responsible management and oversight of these programs to ensure they are safe and effective in disposing of medications.

19. Answer: B

The liability of manufacturers, distributors, and sellers of drugs for harm caused by defective or dangerous products

Explanation: Drug product liability refers to the legal responsibility of those involved in the drug supply chain for harm caused by defective or dangerous drug products.

20. Answer: A

Strict liability

Explanation: Strict liability is a common legal theory used in drug product liability cases when a plaintiff alleges that a drug manufacturer failed to warn about known risks associated with the medication, regardless of whether negligence occurred.

21. **Answer: C**

The manufacturer's failure to adequately warn consumers and healthcare providers about known risks and side effects of a drug

Explanation: "Failure to warn" in a drug product liability case refers to the manufacturer's failure to provide adequate warnings about known risks and side effects of a drug to consumers and healthcare providers.

22. **Answer: B**

Food and Drug Administration (FDA)

Explanation: The FDA regulates drug product labeling and requires manufacturers to include specific information about a drug's risks and benefits on its label.

23. **Answer: C**

To ensure that manufacturers and distributors of drugs produce safe and effective products

Explanation: The primary goal of drug product liability laws and regulations is to ensure that manufacturers and distributors of drugs produce safe and effective products and are held responsible if their products cause harm due to defects or inadequate warnings.

24. **Answer: C**

To identify, mitigate, and prevent risks associated with pharmaceutical products and services

Explanation: The primary purpose of risk management strategies in federal pharmacy law is to identify, mitigate, and prevent risks associated with pharmaceutical products and services to ensure patient safety.

25. Answer: B

Food and Drug Administration (FDA)

Explanation: The FDA is responsible for the development and oversight of risk evaluation and mitigation strategies (REMS) for certain medications to address specific safety concerns.

26. Answer: C

To ensure the safe use of a medication with known risks

Explanation: The primary goal of a REMS program is to ensure the safe use of a medication with known risks by implementing measures to minimize those risks.

27. Answer: B

A patient education document providing essential information about certain prescription medications, typically required when the FDA determines that patient adherence is crucial

Explanation: A Medication Guide is a patient education document that provides essential information about certain prescription medications. It is typically required by the FDA when patient adherence to medication instructions is crucial.

28. Answer: B

Providing medication therapy management (MTM) services

Explanation: Medication therapy management (MTM) services offered by pharmacies are a risk management strategy aimed at preventing medication errors, ensuring proper medication use, and improving patient outcomes.

29. Answer: D

To protect patient health and safety

Explanation: The primary purpose of record-keeping requirements in federal pharmacy law is to protect patient health and safety by ensuring accurate and thorough documentation of pharmacy activities.

30. Answer: A

Drug Enforcement Administration (DEA)

Explanation: The DEA sets and enforces record-keeping requirements for pharmacies related to controlled substances, while other aspects of record-keeping may also fall under the purview of state pharmacy boards.

31. Answer: C

5 years

Explanation: Most pharmacies are required to maintain prescription records for controlled substances for a period of 5 years under federal law.

32. Answer: C

Inventory and drug order records

Explanation: In addition to prescription records, pharmacies are typically required to maintain inventory and drug order records to track the receipt, distribution, and disposition of medications.

33. Answer: D

Loss of DEA registration and ability to handle controlled substances

Explanation: The main consequence for a pharmacy that fails to comply with federal record-keeping requirements, particularly for controlled substances, is the potential loss of its DEA registration, which would result in the inability to handle controlled substances.

34. Answer: A

Drug Enforcement Administration (DEA)

Explanation: The DEA is primarily responsible for the classification and regulation of controlled substances under the Controlled Substances Act (CSA).

35. Answer: A

Schedule I

Explanation: Schedule I substances are considered the most restricted category, with a high potential for abuse and no accepted medical use in the United States.

36. Answer: B

Schedule II

Explanation: Schedule II substances have a high potential for abuse but do have accepted medical uses. They are subject to strict record-keeping and prescription requirements.

37. **Answer: D**

The substance's market demand and pricing

Explanation: Classification of controlled substances is based on factors like potential for abuse, medical use, and safety, but not market demand or pricing.

38. **Answer: C**

To regulate the manufacture, distribution, and dispensing of controlled substances based on their potential for abuse

Explanation: The primary purpose of classifying drugs into schedules is to regulate their handling and distribution based on their potential for abuse and medical use.

39. **Answer: D**

Schedule V

Explanation: Schedule V substances have the lowest potential for abuse and are typically available without a prescription (over-the-counter) under specific conditions.

40. **Answer: D**

Schedule V

Explanation: Codeine-containing cough syrups with non-narcotic ingredients fall under Schedule V when used in specific formulations.

41. **Answer: C**

Schedule III

Explanation: Anabolic steroids used for performance enhancement are classified under Schedule III of controlled substances.

42. **Answer: A**

Drug Enforcement Administration (DEA)

Explanation: The DEA has the authority to reschedule or de-schedule controlled substances based on scientific and medical evaluations.

43. **Answer: D**

Schedule IV

Explanation: Medications like Xanax (alprazolam) and Valium (diazepam) are classified under Schedule IV due to their lower potential for abuse compared to Schedule II and III substances.

44. **Answer: B**

Schedule II

Explanation: Medications like Vicodin (hydrocodone/acetaminophen) and OxyContin (oxycodone) are classified under Schedule II due to their potential for abuse.

45. **Answer: C**

To maintain accurate records of controlled substance transactions

Explanation: Pharmacies must maintain accurate records of controlled substance transactions, including dispensing, receipt, and inventory, as required by federal pharmacy law.

46. Answer: C

Medical doctors (MDs), dentists, and nurse practitioners (NPs)

Explanation: Medical doctors (MDs), dentists, and nurse practitioners (NPs) are typically allowed to prescribe Schedule II controlled substances under certain conditions.

47. Answer: B

The patient must provide written consent for the transfer

Explanation: To transfer a Schedule III or IV prescription from one pharmacy to another, the patient must provide written consent to the transfer.

48. Answer: C

Schedule III

Explanation: Schedule III substances have a moderate potential for abuse and accepted medical use, often with limited refills.

49. Answer: C

The Controlled Substances Act (CSA)

Explanation: The Controlled Substances Act (CSA) established the scheduling system for controlled substances in the United States.

50. Answer: C

Schedule III

Explanation: Medications like Tylenol with codeine are classified under Schedule III of controlled substances.

51. Answer: A

Schedule II medications cannot be refilled, while Schedule III medications can have limited refills

Explanation: Schedule II medications generally cannot be refilled, whereas Schedule III medications can have limited refills with specific requirements.

52. Answer: A

The Controlled Substances Act (CSA)

Explanation: The Controlled Substances Act (CSA) requires pharmacies to maintain separate records for controlled substances and non-controlled substances.

53. Answer: B

The unique registration number issued to healthcare providers and pharmacies by the DEA

Explanation: DEA registration refers to the unique registration number issued by the DEA to healthcare providers and pharmacies, allowing them to handle controlled substances.

54. Answer: C

Schedule III

Explanation: Schedule III controlled substances can be transferred between pharmacies without restrictions, including Schedule II substances, which have more stringent requirements.

55. Answer: C

To ensure that patients have access to needed medications

Explanation: Allowing the transfer of Schedule III, IV, and V controlled substance prescriptions between pharmacies is primarily intended to ensure that patients have access to their needed medications when they move or change pharmacies.

56. Answer: B

Up to three times

Explanation: A prescription for a Schedule III, IV, or V controlled substance can be transferred between pharmacies up to three times, provided that the original prescription has refills available.

57. Answer: C

The date of transfer and the receiving pharmacy's name and address

Explanation: When transferring a Schedule III, IV, or V controlled substance prescription, the transferring pharmacy must document the date of transfer and the name and address of the receiving pharmacy.

58. Answer: A

Transfers are never allowed for Schedule II prescriptions.

Explanation: Schedule II controlled substance prescriptions cannot be transferred between pharmacies under federal law; they must be dispensed directly from the issuing pharmacy.

59. Answer: B

The receiving pharmacist

Explanation: The receiving pharmacist is responsible for ensuring that the patient does not receive more medication than prescribed when a Schedule III, IV, or V controlled substance prescription is transferred.

60. Answer: A

Only when the patient is in a long-term care facilityExplanation: Under federal law, a pharmacy can receive a faxed prescription for a Schedule II controlled substance only when the patient is in a long-term care facility.

61. Answer: C

The pharmacy must obtain the original hard copy of the prescription within 7 days.

Explanation: When a pharmacy receives a faxed prescription for a Schedule II controlled substance, they must obtain the original hard copy of the prescription within 7 days.

62. Answer: C

When the patient is in a long-term care facility or for compound prescriptions

Explanation: Faxed prescriptions for Schedule III, IV, or V controlled substances are allowed when the patient is in a long-term care facility or for compound prescriptions.

63. Answer: C

The prescribing physician's signature

Explanation: A faxed prescription for a controlled substance must include the prescribing physician's signature to be valid under federal law.

5. FEDERAL PHARMACY LAW QUESTIONS PART-5

1. What is the primary purpose of classifying controlled substances into different schedules, including Class II?

    a. To categorize drugs based on their potential for abuse and accepted medical use

    b. To set drug prices in the market

    c. To limit access to certain medications

    d. To regulate the sale of over-the-counter drugs

2. Which federal agency is responsible for overseeing the scheduling of controlled substances in the United States?

    a. FDA (Food and Drug Administration)

    b. CDC (Centers for Disease Control and Prevention)

    c. DEA (Drug Enforcement Administration)

    d. NIH (National Institutes of Health)

3. Which of the following drugs is typically classified as a Class II controlled substance?

    a. Antibiotics

    b. Over-the-counter pain relievers

    c. Methadone

    d. Vitamins

4. What is the key characteristic of Class II controlled substances that distinguishes them from other schedules?

   a. They have a high potential for abuse.

   b. They are available without a prescription.

   c. They can be refilled multiple times.

   d. They are not subject to federal regulations.

5. How often can a prescription for a Class II controlled substance typically be refilled?

   a. As many times as the patient requests

   b. Once, within 72 hours of the original prescription

   c. Never, refills are not allowed

   d. Up to five times within six months

6. What is required on a prescription for a Class II controlled substance to make it valid and legal?

   a. Only the patient's name

   b. Only the prescriber's DEA number

   c. The patient's name, prescriber's signature, and drug name

   d. The pharmacist's signature

7. In the event of theft or loss of a controlled substance, what must a pharmacy do to comply with federal law?

   a. Report the incident to the local police department

   b. Notify the DEA within one business day

   c. Dispose of all controlled substances in the pharmacy

   d. Ignore the incident, as it's a common occurrence

8. How often must pharmacies conduct an inventory of Class II controlled substances?

   a. Weekly

   b. Monthly

   c. Annually

   d. Biennially

9. What is the federal law regarding the transfer of Class II controlled substance prescriptions between pharmacies?

   a. Transfer is not allowed.

   b. Transfers are allowed once.

   c. Transfers are allowed only within the same state.

   d. Transfers are allowed as many times as needed.

10. Which of the following is NOT a requirement for filling a prescription for a Class II controlled substance?

    a. The prescription must be written on tamper-resistant paper.

    b. The pharmacist must record the prescription in a central database.

    c. The pharmacist must verify the prescriber's DEA number.

    d. The patient must provide valid identification.

11. What is the federal requirement for the storage of prescription records for Class II controlled substances?

    a. Must be stored off-site

    b. Must be stored in a secure and retrievable manner

    c. Must be kept indefinitely

    d. Must be shredded after one year

12. How does the federal government classify substances into different schedules, including Class II?

    a. Based solely on their medical use

    b. Based solely on their potential for abuse

    c. Based on a combination of their potential for abuse and medical use

    d. Based on their cost and availability

13. What is the primary purpose of federal regulations surrounding Class II controlled substances?

    a. To generate revenue for the government

    b. To simplify the prescription process for patients

    c. To ensure the safe and secure handling of these substances

    d. To restrict access to necessary medications

14. What information must be included on the label of a dispensed prescription for a Class II controlled substance?

    a. Patient's date of birth

    b. Medication's generic name

    c. Dosage instructions

    d. Refill information

15. What is the role of a pharmacist in verifying the legitimacy of a Class II controlled substance prescription?

    a. Accept all prescriptions without question

    b. Verify the patient's insurance coverage first

    c. Ensure the prescription is valid, including the prescriber's DEA number and patient information

    d. Call the patient to confirm their identity

16. What is the federal law regarding the storage of Class II controlled substances in a pharmacy?

    a. They must be stored in unlocked cabinets for easy access.

    b. They must be stored separately from other medications in a locked cabinet or safe.

    c. They can be stored with non-controlled substances.

    d. They must be stored openly on pharmacy shelves.

17. In which federal schedule are medications with the lowest potential for abuse categorized?

    a. Schedule I

    b. Schedule II

    c. Schedule III

    d. Schedule V

18. What is the federal requirement for documenting the transfer of a Class II controlled substance prescription?

    a. No documentation is needed.

    b. A record of the transfer must be maintained at the transferring pharmacy only.

    c. Both the transferring and receiving pharmacies must maintain records of the transfer.

    d. The patient must sign a waiver for the transfer.

19. What is the purpose of the "closed system" for Class II controlled substances?

    a. To restrict access to these substances to a select group of healthcare providers

    b. To prevent the diversion and abuse of these substances

    c. To allow over-the-counter sales of Class II substances

    d. To eliminate the need for prescription requirements

20. How do federal laws regarding Class II controlled substances impact the practice of telepharmacy?

    a. Telepharmacy is not allowed for Class II substances.

    b. Telepharmacy is only allowed for Class II refills.

    c. Telepharmacy is allowed for Class II prescriptions under specific conditions.

    d. Telepharmacy is exempt from federal regulations.

21. What is misbranding in the context of Federal pharmacy law?

    a. Mixing different medications in the same container

    b. Marketing a generic drug without FDA approval

    c. Providing false or misleading labeling or advertising for a drug

    d. Selling prescription medications without a valid prescription

22. What is the primary purpose of drug labeling according to Federal pharmacy law?

    a. To provide marketing information to healthcare professionals

    b. To make the medication look appealing to patients

    c. To educate patients about the drug's risks and benefits

    d. To increase the price of the medication

23. Which federal agency is responsible for enforcing regulations related to drug labeling and misbranding?

    a. CDC (Centers for Disease Control and Prevention)

    b. DEA (Drug Enforcement Administration)

    c. FDA (Food and Drug Administration)

    d. NIH (National Institutes of Health)

24. What does it mean for a drug to be considered adulterated under Federal pharmacy law?

    a. The drug is counterfeit.

    b. The drug contains an approved ingredient in an incorrect quantity.

    c. The drug is not stored at the correct temperature.

    d. The drug is contaminated or unsafe for use.

25. Which of the following situations would NOT typically lead to a drug being considered adulterated?

    a. Contamination with harmful bacteria during manufacturing

    b. Failure to meet FDA requirements for strength and purity

    c. Having a label that is difficult to read

    d. Misrepresentation of the drug's ingredients on the label

26. What is the primary responsibility of pharmacists regarding misbranded or adulterated drugs in their inventory?

    a. To sell them to consumers at discounted prices

    b. To notify the FDA about the issue

    c. To dispose of them immediately

    d. To continue dispensing them with proper warnings

27. Which type of labeling is required for over-the-counter (OTC) drugs to help consumers use them safely?

    a. Prescription labels

    b. Child-resistant packaging

    c. Drug facts labeling

    d. Expiration date labeling

28. What does the "Rx Only" label on a medication mean?

    a. The medication can only be dispensed with a prescription.

    b. The medication is intended for use by healthcare professionals only.

    c. The medication is not approved by the FDA.

    d. The medication is available without a prescription.

29. Under Federal pharmacy law, what is the role of pharmacists in ensuring that prescription drug labeling is accurate and compliant?

    a. It is not the responsibility of pharmacists.

    b. To create their own labels for prescriptions

    c. To verify the accuracy of prescription labels and make corrections if necessary

    d. To report labeling issues to the patient's insurance company

30. What is the primary purpose of the Drug Listing Act in relation to drug labeling?

    a. To establish pricing guidelines for prescription drugs

    b. To require pharmacies to list their drug inventory online

    c. To create a database of all drugs in commercial distribution

    d. To ban the advertising of prescription medications

31. What federal agency is primarily responsible for regulating the manufacturing and distribution of prescription drugs in the United States?

    a. FDA

    b. DEA

    c. CDC

    d. CMS

32. Which federal law requires pharmacies to maintain patient privacy and confidentiality of medical records?

    a. FDCA

    b. HIPAA

    c. DEA

    d. ACA

33. Under federal law, which schedule of controlled substances has the highest potential for abuse?

    a. Schedule I

    b. Schedule II

    c. Schedule III

    d. Schedule IV

34. Which federal agency enforces laws related to the controlled substances scheduling and registration of prescribers and pharmacies?

    a. FDA

    b. DEA

    c. CMS

    d. CDC

35. The Orange Book is a publication by the FDA that provides information about:

    a. Over-the-counter drugs

    b. Generic drug approvals

    c. Drug recalls

    d. Drug pricing

36. Which federal law requires pharmacies to offer counseling to Medicaid patients and maintain policies for drug utilization review?

    a. HIPAA

    b. FDCA

    c. OBRA '90

    d. CSA

37. Which federal law regulates the compounding of medications by pharmacies and outsourcing facilities?

    a. FDCA

    b. DSHEA

    c. FDAAA

    d. DQSA

38. The Drug Supply Chain Security Act (DSCSA) primarily addresses:

    a. Drug advertising

    b. Drug recalls

    c. Drug importation

    d. Drug traceability

39. Which federal law established the FDA's authority to regulate the marketing and promotion of prescription drugs?

    a. Kefauver-Harris Amendment

    b. Hatch-Waxman Act

    c. Durham-Humphrey Amendment

    d. Prescription Drug User Fee Act (PDUFA)

40. What is the maximum refills allowed for a Schedule III controlled substance prescription under federal law?

    a. 0 refills

    b. 1 refill

    c. 5 refills

    d. Unlimited refills

41. Which federal law established the National Provider Identifier (NPI) and requires healthcare providers, including pharmacists, to obtain one?

    a. HIPAA

    b. FDCA

    c. ACA

    d. DQSA

42. The Federal Food, Drug, and Cosmetic Act (FDCA) primarily focuses on:

    a. Drug scheduling

    b. Drug safety and efficacy

    c. Drug pricing

    d. Drug importation

43. Which federal law requires pharmacies to offer to counsel on the use of prescription medications to all patients?

    a. HIPAA

    b. FDCA

    c. CSA

    d. OBRA '90

44. The federal law that created the Drug Enforcement Administration (DEA) is:

    a. CSA

    b. FDCA

    c. DSCSA

    d. HIPAA

45. Which federal agency is responsible for regulating and overseeing clinical trials for new drugs?

    a. FDA

    b. CDC

    c. NIH

    d. DEA

46. The Drug Price Competition and Patent Term Restoration Act, commonly known as the Hatch-Waxman Act, primarily addresses:

    a. Drug pricing

    b. Generic drug approval

    c. Drug importation

    d. Drug recalls

47. Which of the following is a requirement of the Ryan Haight Online Pharmacy Consumer Protection Act?

    a. Registration of online pharmacies with the DEA

    b. Mandatory counseling for all online prescription orders

    c. A ban on online pharmacies

    d. Mandatory background checks for online pharmacy customers

48. Which federal agency enforces laws related to dietary supplements?

    a. FDA

    b. DEA

    c. CDC

    d. FTC

49. The Federal Anti-Tampering Act primarily addresses:

    a. Drug importation

    b. Drug recalls

    c. Product tampering of consumer goods

    d. Drug pricing

50. Which federal agency is responsible for regulating the labeling and advertising of over-the-counter (OTC) drugs?

    a. FDA

    b. DEA

    c. CDC

    d. FTC

51. The Drug Quality and Security Act (DQSA) was enacted in response to concerns about:

    a. Counterfeit drugs

    b. Drug pricing

    c. Prescription drug abuse

    d. Drug recalls

52. Which federal law established the Prescription Drug Monitoring Program (PDMP) to track controlled substance prescriptions?

    a. CSA

    b. FDCA

    c. DSCSA

    d. DQSA

53. What is the maximum allowed quantity of pseudoephedrine-containing products that can be sold to an individual in a single day without a prescription under federal law?

    a. 3.6 grams

    b. 7.5 grams

    c. 9 grams

    d. 12 grams

54. Which federal agency regulates the labeling and advertising of prescription drugs?

    a. DEA

    b. FTC

    c. FDA

    d. CDC

55. The Dietary Supplement Health and Education Act (DSHEA) primarily:

    a. Regulates dietary supplements as drugs

    b. Regulates dietary supplement manufacturing

    c. Requires dietary supplement prescriptions

    d. Bans dietary supplements

56. Which federal law established a framework for the approval and regulation of biosimilars in the United States?

    a. DSCSA

    b. BPCI Act

    c. Hatch-Waxman Act

    d. FDCA

57. The Orphan Drug Act provides incentives for the development of drugs for rare diseases. What is the designation given to such drugs?

    a. Priority Review

    b. Orphan Drug Designation

    c. Accelerated Approval

    d. Breakthrough Therapy

58. Under the Drug Supply Chain Security Act (DSCSA), which entity is required to provide product tracing information when a prescription drug product is transferred?

    a. Manufacturer

    b. Wholesaler

    c. Pharmacy

    d. Patient

59. Which federal law allows patients to request access to their own medical records and requires healthcare providers to provide them with a copy?

    a. HIPAA

    b. FDCA

    c. DSCSA

    d. BPCI Act

60. Which of the following is NOT a requirement for a prescription to be considered valid under federal law?

    a. A DEA number for controlled substances

    b. The patient's date of birth

    c. The prescriber's signature

    d. The patient's name

61. The Drug Enforcement Administration (DEA) registration is required for:

    a. Patients receiving controlled substances

    b. Pharmacists dispensing controlled substances

    c. Prescribers prescribing controlled substances

    d. All of the above

62. Which federal law established the standards for tamper-evident packaging of over-the-counter (OTC) medications?

    a. FDCA

    b. DEA

    c. DQSA

    d. Federal Anti-Tampering Act

63. The FDA's REMS (Risk Evaluation and Mitigation Strategies) program is primarily aimed at:

    a. Ensuring drug pricing transparency

    b. Monitoring drug recalls

    c. Managing the risks associated with certain medications

    d. Regulating drug importation

64. Which federal law requires pharmacies to maintain records of controlled substance dispensing for at least two years?

    a. CSA

    b. FDCA

    c. DSCSA

    d. OBRA '90

65. Which federal agency oversees the National Drug Code (NDC) system?

    a. FDA

    b. DEA

    c. CDC

    d. FTC

66. What is the primary purpose of the Drug Supply Chain Security Act (DSCSA)?

    a. To regulate drug pricing

    b. To ensure the safety and traceability of the pharmaceutical supply chain

    c. To control drug importation

    d. To monitor drug recalls

67. Which federal law grants pharmacists the authority to administer vaccines to adults?

    a. FDCA

    b. ACA

    c. DSCSA

    d. VFC Program

68. What is the purpose of the Drug Efficacy Study Implementation (DESI) program?

    a. To regulate the importation of drugs

    b. To determine the safety and efficacy of older drugs

    c. To establish the scheduling of controlled substances

    d. To monitor drug recalls

69. Which federal law requires pharmacists to offer to counsel Medicaid patients regarding their prescriptions?

    a. FDCA

    b. HIPAA

    c. ACA

    d. OBRA '90

70. The Drug Price Competition and Patent Term Restoration Act (Hatch-Waxman Act) allows generic drug manufacturers to:

    a. Extend the patent term of branded drugs

    b. Bypass FDA approval for generic drugs

    c. Challenge the patents of brand-name drugs

    d. Set their own prices for generic drugs

71. Under the federal Combat Methamphetamine Epidemic Act, which of the following must be kept behind the pharmacy counter?

    a. Syringes

    b. Birth control pills

    c. Pseudoephedrine-containing products

    d. OTC pain relievers

72. Which federal agency is responsible for regulating the safety and labeling of cosmetics?

    a. FDA

    b. DEA

    c. CDC

    d. FTC

73. The federal law that established the Prescription Drug User Fee Act (PDUFA) allows the FDA to collect fees from:

    a. Drug manufacturers to expedite the drug approval process

    b. Patients to access prescription drug information

    c. Pharmacies to maintain DEA registration

    d. Medicaid beneficiaries

74. Which federal law created the Vaccine Adverse Event Reporting System (VAERS) to monitor the safety of vaccines?

    a. CSA

    b. FDCA

    c. VAERS Act

    d. ACA

75. Which federal agency enforces laws related to the labeling and advertising of tobacco products?

    a. FDA

    b. DEA

    c. CDC

    d. FTC

76. The Dietary Supplement Health and Education Act (DSHEA) allows dietary supplement manufacturers to make health claims on product labels without FDA approval.

    a. True

    b. False

77. Under federal law, who is responsible for ensuring that a prescription is valid and appropriate for the patient's condition?

    a. The patient

    b. The pharmacist

    c. The prescriber

    d. The insurance company

78. Which federal agency regulates the disposal of hazardous waste in healthcare settings, including pharmacies?

    a. FDA

    b. DEA

    c. CDC

    d. EPA

79. Which federal law established the National Vaccine Injury Compensation Program (VICP) to compensate individuals harmed by vaccines?

    a. FDCA

    b. ACA

    c. VICP Act

    d. DSCSA

80. The FDA Amendments Act (FDAAA) introduced a process called Risk Evaluation and Mitigation Strategies (REMS) to:

    a. Streamline the generic drug approval process

    b. Regulate the importation of drugs

    c. Ensure the safe use of certain medications

    d. Control drug pricing

81. What is the primary purpose of the Federal Combat Methamphetamine Epidemic Act (CMEA)?

    a. To regulate the importation of methamphetamine

    b. To combat the illegal production of methamphetamine

    c. To provide treatment for individuals addicted to methamphetamine

    d. To legalize the use of methamphetamine for medical purposes

82. Under the CMEA, which of the following products must be kept behind the pharmacy counter and sold only by a pharmacist or pharmacy technician?

    a. Aspirin

    b. Toothpaste

    c. Pseudoephedrine-containing products

    d. Over-the-counter vitamins

83. What is the maximum amount of pseudoephedrine-containing product that an individual can purchase in a single day under the CMEA without a prescription?

    a. 3 grams

    b. 7.5 grams

    c. 9 grams

    d. 12 grams

84. Which of the following is a requirement of the CMEA for retailers that sell pseudoephedrine-containing products?

    a. Retailers must maintain a logbook of pseudoephedrine sales.

    b. Retailers must provide counseling to customers purchasing these products.

    c. Retailers must refuse to sell any pseudoephedrine products.

    d. Retailers must offer discounts on pseudoephedrine products.

85. Which federal agency is responsible for enforcing the regulations outlined in the Combat Methamphetamine Epidemic Act (CMEA)?

    a. Food and Drug Administration (FDA)

    b. Drug Enforcement Administration (DEA)

    c. Centers for Disease Control and Prevention (CDC)

    d. Federal Trade Commission (FTC)

86. The CMEA requires retailers to verify the identity of purchasers of pseudoephedrine products by:

    a. Collecting a fingerprint

    b. Photocopying the purchaser's driver's license

    c. Scanning the purchaser's retina

    d. Checking a government-issued photo ID and recording the information

87. Which of the following is NOT a requirement for retailers under the CMEA?

    a. Retailers must limit sales to individuals 18 years of age or older.

    b. Retailers must maintain a logbook of sales.

    c. Retailers must provide counseling on the use of pseudoephedrine products.

    d. Retailers must report suspicious sales to the DEA.

88. The CMEA was enacted in response to:

    a. A surge in prescription drug abuse

    b. A rise in methamphetamine production and abuse

    c. A shortage of cold and allergy medications

    d. An increase in tobacco use

89. Which of the following individuals is exempt from the purchase restrictions on pseudoephedrine products under the CMEA?

    a. Anyone under the age of 21

    b. Individuals with a valid prescription

    c. Foreign tourists

    d. Retail employees

90. The CMEA imposes civil and criminal penalties for violations, including fines and imprisonment. Violations can result in penalties for:

    a. Retailers and purchasers

    b. Retailers only

    c. Purchasers only

    d. Manufacturers of pseudoephedrine products

91. What is the primary purpose of a Federal Pharmacy Patient Package Insert (PPI)?

    a. To provide dosage instructions to healthcare providers

    b. To contain pricing information for medications

    c. To offer comprehensive information to patients about their medications

    d. To track the expiration date of pharmaceutical products

92. Which federal agency mandates the inclusion of PPIs with certain prescription medications?

    a. Drug Enforcement Administration (DEA)

    b. Centers for Disease Control and Prevention (CDC)

    c. Food and Drug Administration (FDA)

    d. National Institutes of Health (NIH)

93. What information is typically included in a PPI?

    a. Manufacturer's contact information only

    b. Medication name and dosage form only

    c. Dosage instructions, side effects, warnings, and other essential information

    d. Prescription pricing and insurance details only

94. When should a pharmacist provide a PPI to a patient?

    a. Only upon patient request

    b. At the pharmacist's discretion

    c. With every prescription medication, both new and refill orders

    d. Only for controlled substances

95. Which of the following is NOT typically found in a PPI?

    a. Dosage instructions

    b. Manufacturer's contact information

    c. Information on how to store the medication

    d. Prescription pricing and insurance coverage details

96. What is the primary purpose of a Risk Evaluation and Mitigation Strategy (REMS) mandated by the FDA?

    a. To promote the sales and marketing of pharmaceutical products

    b. To facilitate the importation of specialty drugs

    c. To ensure the safe use of certain medications with known risks

    d. To streamline the approval process for generic drugs

97. Which federal agency is responsible for requiring REMS programs for specific medications?

    a. Drug Enforcement Administration (DEA)

    b. Centers for Disease Control and Prevention (CDC)

    c. Food and Drug Administration (FDA)

    d. National Institutes of Health (NIH)

98. What components are typically included in a REMS program?

    a. Only medication pricing information

    b. Patient education, prescriber certification, dispensing restrictions, and more

    c. Manufacturer's contact information

    d. Prescription drug importation details

99. When is a REMS program typically required for a medication?

    a. Only for over-the-counter (OTC) medications

    b. When the medication is first approved by the FDA

    c. For all medications on the market

    d. When the medication's patent expires

100. Which of the following is NOT a goal of a REMS program?

a. To enhance patient access to medications

b. To ensure the safe use of medications

c. To minimize the risks associated with certain drugs

d. To prevent medication-related adverse events

5. FEDERAL PHARMACY LAW ANSWERS PART-5

1. **Answer: A**

   To categorize drugs based on their potential for abuse and accepted medical use.

   Explanation: The classification helps in regulating their handling and distribution.

2. **Answer: C**

   DEA (Drug Enforcement Administration).

   Explanation: The DEA is responsible for regulating controlled substances, including scheduling.

3. **Answer: C**

   Methadone.

   Explanation: Methadone is an example of a Class II controlled substance used to treat opioid addiction.

4. **Answer: A**

   They have a high potential for abuse.

   Explanation: Class II controlled substances are known for their high potential for abuse and dependence.

5. **Answer: C**

   Never, refills are not allowed.

   Explanation: In general, Class II controlled substances do not permit refills.

6. **Answer: C**

The patient's name, prescriber's signature, and drug name.

Explanation: A valid prescription for a Class II controlled substance must include these essential elements.

7. **Answer: B**

Notify the DEA within one business day.

Explanation: Federal law requires pharmacies to report theft or loss of controlled substances to the DEA promptly.

8. **Answer: C**

Annually.

Explanation: Pharmacies are required to conduct an annual inventory of Class II controlled substances.

9. **Answer: B**

Explanation: Transfers are allowed once between pharmacies, under specific conditions and requirements.

10. **Answer: B**

The pharmacist must record the prescription in a central database.

Explanation: While some states have prescription monitoring programs, this is not a federal requirement for filling a Class II prescription.

11. **Answer: B**

Must be stored in a secure and retrievable manner.

Explanation: Prescription records for Class II controlled substances must be securely maintained for a specified period.

12. **Answer: C**

Based on a combination of their potential for abuse and medical use.

Explanation: Federal scheduling considers both the potential for abuse and accepted medical use.

13. **Answer: C**

To ensure the safe and secure handling of these substances.

Explanation: Federal regulations aim to prevent diversion and misuse of Class II controlled substances.

14. **Answer: B**

Medication's generic name.

Explanation: The label on dispensed prescription medications should include the medication's generic name, among other information.

15. **Answer: C**

Ensure the prescription is valid, including the prescriber's DEA number and patient information.

Explanation: Pharmacists must verify the legitimacy of Class II prescriptions.

16. **Answer: B**

They must be stored separately from other medications in a locked cabinet or safe.

Explanation: Class II controlled substances must be securely stored separately.

17. **Answer: D**

Schedule V.

Explanation: Schedule V substances have the lowest potential for abuse among controlled substances.

18. **Answer: C**

Both the transferring and receiving pharmacies must maintain records of the transfer.

Explanation: Documentation is required at both pharmacies involved in the transfer.

19. **Answer: B**

To prevent the diversion and abuse of these substances.

Explanation: The closed system aims to control and track Class II substances to prevent misuse.

20. **Answer: C**

Telepharmacy is allowed for Class II prescriptions under specific conditions.

Explanation: Telepharmacy may be used for Class II prescriptions as long as federal and state regulations are followed, including identity verification and record-keeping.

21. **Answer: C**

Providing false or misleading labeling or advertising for a drug.

Explanation: Misbranding occurs when a drug's labeling or advertising is inaccurate or deceptive.

22. **Answer: C**

To educate patients about the drug's risks and benefits.

Explanation: Drug labeling is intended to inform patients and healthcare professionals about a drug's proper use and potential risks.

23. **Answer: C**

FDA (Food and Drug Administration).

Explanation: The FDA is responsible for enforcing regulations related to drug labeling and misbranding.

24. **Answer: D**

The drug is contaminated or unsafe for use.

Explanation: An adulterated drug is one that does not meet safety and quality standards.

25. **Answer: C**

Having a label that is difficult to read.

Explanation: While clear labeling is essential for patient safety, it does not typically result in a drug being considered adulterated.

26. **Answer: C**

To dispose of them immediately.

Explanation: Pharmacists should not dispense misbranded or adulterated drugs and should follow proper disposal procedures.

27. **Answer: C**

Drug facts labeling.

Explanation: OTC drugs must have drug facts labeling to provide consumers with information on proper use and potential risks.

28. **Answer: A**

The medication can only be dispensed with a prescription.

Explanation: The "Rx Only" label indicates that the medication requires a prescription.

29. **Answer: C**

To verify the accuracy of prescription labels and make corrections if necessary.

Explanation: Pharmacists play a crucial role in ensuring that prescription labels are accurate and compliant with federal regulations.

30. **Answer: C**

To create a database of all drugs in commercial distribution.

Explanation: The Drug Listing Act requires drug manufacturers and distributors to submit information about their products to the FDA's National Drug Code Directory. This helps maintain an accurate database of all drugs in commercial distribution.

31. **Answer: A**

FDA

Explanation: The Food and Drug Administration (FDA) is responsible for regulating prescription drugs' manufacturing and distribution.

32. **Answer: B**

HIPAA

Explanation: The Health Insurance Portability and Accountability Act (HIPAA) mandates patient privacy and confidentiality.

33. **Answer: A**

Schedule I

Explanation: Schedule I substances have the highest potential for abuse and are illegal for most purposes.

34. **Answer: B**

DEA

Explanation: The Drug Enforcement Administration (DEA) enforces controlled substance laws and regulations.

35. **Answer: B**

Generic drug approvals

Explanation: The Orange Book lists approved generic drugs and their therapeutic equivalence to brand-name drugs.

36. **Answer: C**

OBRA '90

Explanation: The Omnibus Budget Reconciliation Act of 1990 (OBRA '90) mandates counseling for Medicaid patients and drug utilization review.

37. Answer: D

DQSA

Explanation: The Drug Quality and Security Act (DQSA) regulates compounding by pharmacies and outsourcing facilities.

38. Answer: D

Drug traceability

Explanation: DSCSA focuses on ensuring the traceability and security of the pharmaceutical supply chain.

39. Answer: A

Kefauver-Harris Amendment

Explanation: The Kefauver-Harris Amendment gave the FDA authority to regulate drug marketing and promotion.

40. Answer: C

5 Refills

Explanation: Federal law allows up to 5 refills for Schedule III controlled substances within 6 months.

41. Answer: A

HIPAA

Explanation: HIPAA established the NPI system and mandates its use for healthcare providers.

42. **Answer: B**

Drug safety and efficacy

Explanation: The FDCA primarily addresses drug safety and efficacy.

43. **Answer: D**

OBRA '90

Explanation: OBRA '90 mandates offering counseling on prescription drug use to all patients.

44. **Answer: A**

CSA

Explanation: The Controlled Substances Act (CSA) established the DEA.

45. **Answer: A**

FDA

Explanation: The FDA oversees and regulates clinical trials for new drugs.

46. **Answer: B**

Generic drug approval

Explanation: The Hatch-Waxman Act streamlines the approval process for generic drugs.

47. **Answer: A**

Registration of online pharmacies with the DEA

Explanation: The Ryan Haight Act requires online pharmacies to register with the DEA.

48. **Answer: A**

FDA

Explanation: The FDA regulates dietary supplements in the United States.

49. **Answer: C**

Product tampering of consumer goods

Explanation: The Federal Anti-Tampering Act addresses tampering with consumer products.

50. **Answer: A**

FDA

Explanation: The FDA regulates the labeling and advertising of OTC drugs.

51. **Answer: A**

Counterfeit drugs

Explanation: DQSA addresses concerns about counterfeit drugs and the safety of the drug supply.

52. **Answer: A**

CSA

Explanation: The Controlled Substances Act (CSA) laid the foundation for PDMPs.

53. **Answer: B**

7.5 grams

Explanation: Federal law limits non-prescription sales of pseudoephedrine-containing products to 7.5 grams per day.

54. **Answer: C**

FDA

Explanation: The FDA regulates the labeling and advertising of prescription drugs.

55. **Answer: B**

Regulates dietary supplement manufacturing

Explanation: DSHEA primarily regulates the manufacturing of dietary supplements.

56. **Answer: B**

BPCI Act

Explanation: The Biologics Price Competition and Innovation (BPCI) Act addresses biosimilar approval and regulation.

57. **Answer: B**

Orphan Drug Designation

Explanation: The Orphan Drug Act provides orphan drug designation to incentivize rare disease drug development.

58. **Answer: B**

Wholesaler

Explanation: Wholesalers are required to provide product tracing information under DSCSA.

59. **Answer: A**

HIPAA

Explanation: HIPAA allows patients to request access to their medical records.

60. **Answer: B**

The patient's date of birth

Explanation: The patient's date of birth is not required on a prescription.

61. **Answer: D**

All of the above

Explanation: DEA registration is required for patients, pharmacists, and prescribers involved with controlled substances.

62. **Answer: D**

Federal Anti-Tampering Act

Explanation: The Federal Anti-Tampering Act sets standards for tamper-evident packaging of OTC drugs.

63. **Answer: C**

Managing the risks associated with certain medications

Explanation: REMS is designed to manage the risks associated with specific drugs.

64. **Answer: A**

CSA

Explanation: The Controlled Substances Act (CSA) mandates record-keeping for controlled substances.

65. **Answer: A**

FDA

Explanation: The FDA oversees the NDC system, which identifies drugs.

66. **Answer: B**

To ensure the safety and traceability of the pharmaceutical supply chain

Explanation: DSCSA's primary purpose is to ensure the safety and traceability of the pharmaceutical supply chain.

67. **Answer: B**

ACA

Explanation: The Affordable Care Act (ACA) grants pharmacists the authority to administer vaccines to adults.

68. **Answer: B**

To determine the safety and efficacy of older drugs

Explanation: The DESI program evaluates the safety and efficacy of older drugs.

69. **Answer: D**

OBRA '90

Explanation: OBRA '90 mandates counseling for Medicaid patients.

70. **Answer: C**

Challenge the patents of brand-name drugs

Explanation: The Hatch-Waxman Act allows generic drug manufacturers to challenge the patents of brand-name drugs.

71. **Answer: C**

Pseudoephedrine-containing products

Explanation: The Combat Methamphetamine Epidemic Act requires pseudoephedrine products to be kept behind the pharmacy counter.

72. **Answer: A**

FDA

Explanation: The FDA regulates the safety and labeling of cosmetics.

73. **Answer: A**

Drug manufacturers to expedite the drug approval process

Explanation: PDUFA allows the FDA to collect fees from drug manufacturers to expedite drug approvals.

74. **Answer: C**

VAERS Act

Explanation: The VAERS Act established the Vaccine Adverse Event Reporting System.

75. **Answer: A**

FDA

Explanation: The FDA regulates the labeling and advertising of tobacco products.

76. **Answer: A**

True

Explanation: DSHEA allows dietary supplement manufacturers to make certain health claims without FDA preapproval.

77. **Answer: B**

The pharmacist

Explanation: Pharmacists are responsible for ensuring the validity and appropriateness of prescriptions.

78. **Answer: D**

EPA

Explanation: The Environmental Protection Agency (EPA) regulates the disposal of hazardous waste in healthcare settings.

79. **Answer: C**

VICP Act

Explanation: The VICP Act established the National Vaccine Injury Compensation Program.

80. **Answer: C**

Ensure the safe use of certain medications

Explanation: FDAAA introduced REMS to ensure the safe use of specific medications.

81. **Answer: B**

To combat the illegal production of methamphetamine

Explanation: The CMEA was enacted to combat the illegal production of methamphetamine by regulating the sale of pseudoephedrine-containing products, which are commonly used in the manufacturing of methamphetamine.

82. **Answer: C**

Pseudoephedrine-containing products

Explanation: The CMEA requires that products containing pseudoephedrine, such as cold and allergy medications, be kept behind the pharmacy counter and sold only by pharmacy staff.

83. **Answer: B**

7.5 grams

Explanation: The CMEA limits non-prescription sales of pseudoephedrine-containing products to 7.5 grams per day per individual.

84. Answer: A

Retailers must maintain a logbook of pseudoephedrine sales.

Explanation: The CMEA mandates that retailers selling pseudoephedrine-containing products must maintain a logbook to track sales, including purchaser information.

85. Answer: B

Drug Enforcement Administration (DEA)

Explanation: The DEA is responsible for enforcing the regulations related to pseudoephedrine-containing products under the CMEA.

86. Answer: D

Checking a government-issued photo ID and recording the information

Explanation: Retailers are required to check a government-issued photo ID, such as a driver's license, and record the purchaser's information when selling pseudoephedrine products.

87. Answer: C

Retailers must provide counseling on the use of pseudoephedrine products.

Explanation: While retailers are required to maintain a logbook and report suspicious sales, they are not required to provide counseling on the use of pseudoephedrine products under the CMEA.

88. Answer: B

A rise in methamphetamine production and abuse

Explanation: The CMEA was enacted to address the increase in methamphetamine production and abuse, particularly related to the diversion of pseudoephedrine-containing products.

89. Answer: B

Individuals with a valid prescription

Explanation: Individuals with a valid prescription for pseudoephedrine products are exempt from the purchase restrictions under the CMEA.

90. Answer: A

Retailers and purchasers

Explanation: The CMEA imposes penalties for both retailers and purchasers who violate its regulations, including fines and imprisonment.

91. Answer: C

To offer comprehensive information to patients about their medications

Explanation: The primary purpose of a PPI is to provide patients with essential information about their medications, including proper usage, side effects, and precautions.

92. Answer: C

Food and Drug Administration (FDA)

Explanation: The FDA mandates the inclusion of PPIs with certain prescription medications to ensure that patients receive critical information about their drugs.

93. Answer: C

Dosage instructions, side effects, warnings, and other essential information

Explanation: PPIs typically include dosage instructions, side effects, warnings, precautions, and other crucial information to help patients use their medications safely and effectively.

94. Answer: C

With every prescription medication, both new and refill orders

Explanation: Pharmacists are generally required to provide a PPI with every prescription medication, whether it's a new prescription or a refill, to ensure patients have access to essential drug information.

95. Answer: D

Prescription pricing and insurance coverage details

Explanation: PPIs typically do not contain information about prescription pricing or insurance coverage details. Their focus is on medication usage and safety information for patients.

96. Answer: C

To ensure the safe use of certain medications with known risks

Explanation: The primary purpose of a REMS is to mitigate known risks associated with certain medications and ensure their safe use by patients.

97. Answer: C

Food and Drug Administration (FDA)

Explanation: The FDA is responsible for mandating REMS programs for specific medications, particularly those with known safety concerns.

98. Answer: B

Patient education, prescriber certification, dispensing restrictions, and more

Explanation: REMS programs typically include multiple components, such as patient education, prescriber certification, dispensing restrictions, and more, to manage medication risks.

99. Answer: B

When the medication is first approved by the FDA

Explanation: REMS programs are usually required when a medication is initially approved by the FDA or when new safety concerns arise during its post-approval period.

100. Answer: A

To enhance patient access to medications

Explanation: While REMS programs aim to ensure the safe use of medications and minimize risks, their primary goal is not to enhance patient access. In some cases, REMS may include restrictions on access to ensure safe use.

6. FEDERAL PHARMACY LAW QUESTIONS PART-6

1. Who has the primary responsibility for initiating a recall of a pharmaceutical product in the United States?

   a. The FDA

   b. The manufacturer or distributor

   c. The pharmacy

   d. The prescribing healthcare provider

2. Which federal agency oversees and enforces pharmaceutical recalls in the United States?

   a. Drug Enforcement Administration (DEA)

   b. Centers for Disease Control and Prevention (CDC)

   c. Food and Drug Administration (FDA)

   d. National Institutes of Health (NIH)

3. What is the primary reason for initiating a Class I pharmaceutical recall?

   a. To correct a minor labeling error

   b. To retrieve expired medications from the market

   c. To address a defect that could cause serious harm or death

   d. To reduce production costs

4. When a pharmacy receives notice of a drug recall, what is the most important initial action they should take?

   a. Continue dispensing the recalled product until it runs out of stock

   b. Quarantine the recalled product and stop dispensing it immediately

   c. Ignore the recall notice if the product is already in patients' hands

   d. Contact the prescribing healthcare provider for guidance

5. Which of the following is NOT a recommended step in handling a pharmaceutical recall at a pharmacy?

   a. Notify patients who have received the recalled product

   b. Document all actions related to the recall

   c. Wait for the FDA to provide instructions before taking any action

   d. Return the recalled product to the manufacturer or distributor

6. Which category of controlled substances includes medications with a moderate to low potential for physical and psychological dependence?

   a. Schedule I

   b. Schedule II

   c. Schedule III

   d. Schedule IV

7. Under federal law, which of the following healthcare providers can prescribe Schedule III and IV controlled substances?

   a. Physicians only

   b. Nurse practitioners and physician assistants

   c. Pharmacists

   d. Dentists only

8. What is the maximum allowable refill quantity for a Schedule III or IV controlled substance prescription under federal law?

   a. No refills allowed

   b. One refill

   c. Five refills within 6 months

   d. Unlimited refills

9. What is the typical duration of a Schedule III or IV controlled substance prescription, as allowed by federal law?

   a. 7 days

   b. 14 days

   c. 30 days

   d. 90 days

10. Which federal agency enforces the regulations surrounding Schedule III and IV controlled substances?

    a. Drug Enforcement Administration (DEA)

    b. Food and Drug Administration (FDA)

    c. Centers for Disease Control and Prevention (CDC)

    d. National Institutes of Health (NIH)

11. Which of the following is NOT a common Schedule IV controlled substance?

    a. Alprazolam (Xanax)

    b. Lorazepam (Ativan)

    c. Hydrocodone (Vicodin)

    d. Zolpidem (Ambien)

12. What is the primary factor that determines a controlled substance's placement into a specific schedule?

    a. Its potential for abuse

    b. Its cost

    c. Its chemical composition

    d. Its expiration date

13. Which schedule includes controlled substances with a high potential for abuse and no accepted medical use in the United States?

    a. Schedule I

    b. Schedule II

    c. Schedule III

    d. Schedule IV

14. What is the primary purpose of scheduling controlled substances into different categories (schedules)?

    a. To set maximum allowable prices for medications

    b. To facilitate international drug trade

    c. To regulate the manufacturing and distribution of controlled substances

    d. To increase the availability of medications to patients

15. Which of the following healthcare professionals can dispense Schedule III and IV controlled substances to patients?

    a. Pharmacists only

    b. Physicians only

    c. Dentists only

    d. Nurse practitioners, physician assistants, and pharmacists

16. According to federal law, how many times can a Schedule III to V prescription be transferred between pharmacies?

    a. Once

    b. Twice

    c. Three times

    d. An unlimited number of times

17. Which of the following healthcare professionals can initiate the transfer of a Schedule III to V prescription?

    a. Only the prescribing physician

    b. Pharmacists and pharmacy technicians

    c. Nurse practitioners and physician assistants

    d. All of the above

18. When transferring a Schedule III to V prescription, which piece of information is NOT typically required on the prescription transfer record?

    a. Name of the receiving pharmacy

    b. Date of the transfer

    c. Name of the pharmacist at the receiving pharmacy

    d. National Provider Identifier (NPI) of the prescribing healthcare provider

19. What is the maximum allowable time frame for completing the transfer of a Schedule III to V prescription, including the initial dispense?

    a. 7 days

    b. 14 days

    c. 30 days

    d. 90 days

20. What information must be communicated to the receiving pharmacy when transferring a Schedule III to V prescription?

    a. Only the prescription number

    b. Only the patient's name

    c. Prescription number, patient's name, and the quantity dispensed

    d. Prescription number, patient's name, and the prescriber's name

21. In which schedule category does a medication with a moderate potential for abuse and accepted medical use fall?

    a. Schedule I

    b. Schedule II

    c. Schedule III

    d. Schedule IV

22. What is the primary federal law that governs the transfer of Schedule III to V prescriptions between pharmacies?

    a. The Controlled Substances Act (CSA)

    b. The Food, Drug, and Cosmetic Act (FDCA)

    c. The Affordable Care Act (ACA)

    d. The Poison Prevention Packaging Act (PPPA)

23. Which federal agency is responsible for enforcing the regulations related to controlled substances and prescription transfers?

    a. Drug Enforcement Administration (DEA)

    b. Centers for Medicare & Medicaid Services (CMS)

    c. Food and Drug Administration (FDA)

    d. National Institutes of Health (NIH)

24. What is the maximum allowable quantity of a Schedule III to V controlled substance that can be transferred between pharmacies?

    a. One day's supply

    b. A 72-hour supply

    c. A 30-day supply

    d. A 90-day supply

25. Under federal law, what is the minimum age requirement for a pharmacy technician to participate in the transfer of Schedule III to V prescriptions?

    a. 16 years old

    b. 18 years old

    c. 21 years old

    d. There is no minimum age requirement

26. Which federal program provides healthcare coverage primarily for individuals aged 65 and older, as well as some younger individuals with certain disabilities?

    a. Medicare

    b. Medicaid

    c. CHIP

    d. TRICARE

27. What is the primary federal agency responsible for administering the Medicare program?

    a. Centers for Disease Control and Prevention (CDC)

    b. Drug Enforcement Administration (DEA)

    c. Centers for Medicare & Medicaid Services (CMS)

    d. Food and Drug Administration (FDA)

28. Which part of Medicare covers prescription drug benefits for Medicare beneficiaries?

    a. Medicare Part A

    b. Medicare Part B

    c. Medicare Part C

    d. Medicare Part D

29. Medicaid is a joint federal and state program that provides healthcare coverage primarily for:

    a. Individuals aged 65 and older

    b. Low-income individuals and families

    c. Active-duty military personnel

    d. Veterans

30. Which federal agency oversees the Medicaid program and sets certain federal regulations and guidelines?

    a. Drug Enforcement Administration (DEA)

    b. Centers for Disease Control and Prevention (CDC)

    c. Centers for Medicare & Medicaid Services (CMS)

    d. Food and Drug Administration (FDA)

31. Which federal law expanded Medicaid eligibility to include more low-income adults in participating states?

    a. Social Security Act

    b. Affordable Care Act (ACA)

    c. Medicare Modernization Act (MMA)

    d. Medicaid Expansion Act

32. Pharmacies that participate in Medicare Part D must adhere to which set of regulations governing prescription drug coverage and claims processing?

    a. HIPAA regulations

    b. FDA regulations

    c. Medicare Part B regulations

    d. Medicare Part D regulations

33. Which of the following is NOT a factor considered when determining eligibility for Medicaid?

    a. Income

    b. Age

    c. Disability status

    d. Citizenship or immigration status

34. Which program provides healthcare coverage for low-income children in the United States?

    a. Medicare

    b. Medicaid

    c. CHIP

    d. TRICARE

35. What is the primary purpose of the Drug Utilization Review (DUR) program within Medicaid?

    a. To increase the cost of prescription medications

    b. To limit access to prescription drugs

    c. To ensure the safe and effective use of prescription medications

    d. To eliminate prescription drug coverage

36. Which federal agency is primarily responsible for regulating and enforcing laws related to controlled substances, including prescription medications with potential for abuse?

    a. Food and Drug Administration (FDA)

    b. Centers for Disease Control and Prevention (CDC)

    c. Drug Enforcement Administration (DEA)

    d. National Institutes of Health (NIH)

37. What is the primary mission of the DEA regarding controlled substances?

    a. To promote the pharmaceutical industry

    b. To reduce the availability of controlled substances

    c. To oversee clinical trials of new drugs

    d. To regulate the pricing of prescription medications

38. Which federal agency is responsible for approving new drugs for marketing in the United States and ensuring their safety and efficacy?

    a. Drug Enforcement Administration (DEA)

    b. Centers for Disease Control and Prevention (CDC)

    c. Food and Drug Administration (FDA)

    d. National Institutes of Health (NIH)

39. What is the primary purpose of the FDA's Center for Drug Evaluation and Research (CDER)?

    a. To regulate food products

    b. To evaluate and approve new drugs

    c. To enforce controlled substance laws

    d. To regulate the importation of medical devices

40. What is the FDA's role in the regulation of dietary supplements?

    a. The FDA does not regulate dietary supplements.

    b. The FDA strictly enforces regulations on dietary supplements.

    c. The FDA approves all dietary supplements before they can be sold.

    d. The FDA sets maximum pricing for dietary supplements.

41. Which federal agency is responsible for tracking and investigating outbreaks of foodborne illnesses and ensuring the safety of the food supply?

    a. Drug Enforcement Administration (DEA)

    b. Centers for Disease Control and Prevention (CDC)

    c. Food and Drug Administration (FDA)

    d. National Institutes of Health (NIH)

42. What is the primary function of the FDA's Center for Biologics Evaluation and Research (CBER)?

    a. To regulate veterinary medications

    b. To oversee the safety of vaccines and blood products

    c. To enforce drug importation laws

    d. To conduct clinical trials of new drugs

43. The Drug Enforcement Administration (DEA) assigns a unique registration number to:

   a. Pharmaceutical manufacturers

   b. Pharmacists

   c. Patients

   d. Prescribing healthcare providers

44. What is the primary purpose of the FDA's MedWatch program?

   a. To regulate the importation of medical devices

   b. To track adverse events and safety concerns related to medications and medical products

   c. To conduct clinical trials of new drugs

   d. To enforce food safety regulations

45. Which federal agency is responsible for regulating the labeling and advertising of tobacco products?

   a. Drug Enforcement Administration (DEA)

   b. Centers for Disease Control and Prevention (CDC)

   c. Food and Drug Administration (FDA)

   d. National Institutes of Health (NIH)

46. Which federal agency is primarily responsible for regulating medication development and marketing in the United States?

    a. DEA

    b. CDC

    c. FDA

    d. NIH

47. What does the acronym "DEA" stand for in the context of pharmacy law?

    a. Drug Enforcement Administration

    b. Drug Evaluation Agency

    c. Drug Enforcement Act

    d. Drug Expiration Agenc.

48. Which of the following is a key requirement for a drug to be classified as an over-the-counter (OTC) medication?

    a. Prescription-only status

    b. Available without a prescription

    c. Requires a physician's referral

    d. Available only to certain age groups

49. What does the Hatch-Waxman Act primarily relate to in the pharmaceutical industry?

    a. Drug pricing regulations

    b. Generic drug approval

    c. Drug patent extensions

    d. Drug manufacturing standards

50. What are REMS (Risk Evaluation and Mitigation Strategies) designed to address?

    a. Generic drug safety

    b. OTC medication labeling

    c. Medication advertising

    d. Risk management for certain medications

51. How does the FDA regulate the advertising and promotion of prescription drugs?

    a. It has no authority over drug advertising.

    b. It reviews and approves all drug advertisements.

    c. It enforces regulations to ensure accurate and balanced drug promotion.

    d. It relies solely on pharmaceutical companies to self-regulate advertising.

52. What is the primary purpose of the Orphan Drug Act?

a. To regulate drug importation

b. To encourage the development of medications for rare diseases

c. To regulate drug pricing

d. To promote generic drug competition

53. What do Good Manufacturing Practices (GMPs) primarily focus on in the pharmaceutical industry?

a. Drug pricing

b. Medication safety

c. Drug advertising

d. Drug importation

54. What are biosimilars in the context of medication regulation?

a. Identical copies of brand-name drugs

b. Generic versions of biologic drugs

c. Specialty medications

d. OTC medications

55. How does the Federal Anti-Tampering Act protect the integrity of over-the-counter medications?

a. It regulates the pricing of OTC medications.

b. It ensures the safety of OTC medication ingredients.

c. It addresses tampering and contamination issues with OTC products.

d. It mandates prescription-only status for OTC medications.

56. What role does the Federal Trade Commission (FTC) play in regulating medication advertising and marketing?

a. It approves all medication advertisements.

b. It enforces antitrust laws within the pharmaceutical industry.

c. It oversees medication manufacturing standards.

d. It reviews and approves medication labels.

57. What is the main focus of the Drug Supply Chain Security Act (DSCSA)?

a. Regulating drug prices

b. Ensuring medication accessibility

c. Enhancing medication safety and tracing

d. Promoting pharmaceutical advertising

58. Which federal agency primarily regulates the approval and oversight of biologic drugs in the United States?

a. Drug Enforcement Administration (DEA)

b. Federal Trade Commission (FTC)

c. Food and Drug Administration (FDA)

d. Centers for Disease Control and Prevention (CDC)

59. What distinguishes biologic drugs from traditional small-molecule drugs?

a. Biologics are always administered orally.

b. Biologics are synthesized through chemical processes.

c. Biologics are typically derived from living organisms.

d. Biologics have a longer shelf life.

60. What is the regulatory pathway for the approval of biosimilars in the United States?

a. Abbreviated New Drug Application (ANDA)

b. Biologics License Application (BLA)

c. New Drug Application (NDA)

d. Investigational New Drug Application (IND)

61. What role does the Purple Book play in the regulation of biologic drugs?

a. It provides information on drug pricing.

b. It lists approved biosimilar products.

c. It regulates drug advertising.

d. It addresses drug importation issues.

62. What does the Biologics Price Competition and Innovation Act (BPCIA) aim to achieve?

a. Regulating drug importation

b. Promoting the development of biosimilars

c. Ensuring drug accessibility

d. Regulating pharmaceutical advertising

63. What federal agency regulates and sets guidelines for the content and format of prescription drug labeling information for the patient?

a. Drug Enforcement Administration (DEA)

b. Federal Trade Commission (FTC)

c. Food and Drug Administration (FDA)

d. Centers for Disease Control and Prevention (CDC)

64. Which of the following is typically NOT included in the "Patient Information" section of prescription drug labeling?

a. Dosage instructions

b. Potential side effects

c. Information on the drug's manufacturer

d. How to store the medication

65. What is the purpose of the "Black Box Warning" in prescription drug labeling?

a. To highlight the drug's brand name

b. To emphasize the potential for severe or life-threatening side effects

c. To indicate the drug's expiration date

d. To list all possible drug interactions

66. Which of the following statements is true regarding the "Instructions for Use" section of prescription drug labeling?

a. It provides information for healthcare professionals only.

b. It offers guidance on how to administer the drug to patients.

c. It includes pricing information for the medication.

d. It is optional and not required by the FDA.

67. In the United States, what is the standard format for the "Drug Facts" label on over-the-counter (OTC) medications?

    a. The Physician Package Insert (PPI)
    b. The Medication Guide (MedGuide)
    c. The Prescription Drug Label (PDL)
    d. The Drug Facts panel

68. What is the primary distinction between pharmacy compounding and drug manufacturing?

    a. Compounding is performed by pharmacists, while manufacturing is done by pharmaceutical companies.
    b. Compounding is always done on a large scale, while manufacturing is typically small-scale.
    c. Compounding involves the creation of new drug formulations, while manufacturing produces existing drugs.
    d. Compounding is regulated by state pharmacy boards, while manufacturing is regulated by the FDA.

69. Which federal law specifically outlines the regulatory framework for pharmacy compounding?

    a. Federal Food, Drug, and Cosmetic Act (FDCA)
    b. Drug Quality and Security Act (DQSA)
    c. Controlled Substances Act (CSA)
    d. Dietary Supplement Health and Education Act (DSHEA)

70. What is the role of the United States Pharmacopeia (USP) in pharmacy compounding?

   a. USP sets standards for the manufacturing of commercial drugs.

   b. USP provides guidance for pharmacy compounding practices.

   c. USP enforces regulations for controlled substances.

   d. USP approves drug advertising.

71. Which of the following statements is true regarding the outsourcing of pharmacy compounding?

   a. Outsourcing compounding facilities are subject to the same regulations as traditional pharmacies.

   b. Outsourcing compounding facilities are not regulated by any federal agency.

   c. Outsourcing compounding facilities are exempt from all compounding regulations.

   d. Outsourcing compounding facilities are regulated solely by state pharmacy boards.

72. When does the FDA exercise its authority to regulate compounding pharmacies more like drug manufacturers?

   a. When a compounding pharmacy operates in multiple states

   b. When a compounding pharmacy uses bulk drug substances that are not on an FDA-approved list

   c. When a compounding pharmacy provides compounded medications for individual patient prescriptions only

   d. When a compounding pharmacy is a member of a professional pharmacy association

73. What is the "Orange Book" in the context of federal pharmacy law?

a. A reference book for prescription drug pricing information

b. A publication listing generic drug products and their equivalence to brand-name drugs

c. A regulatory document outlining drug manufacturing standards

d. A database of over-the-counter (OTC) medications

74. What does the term "AB rating" indicate in the Orange Book?

a. It signifies that a generic drug product is therapeutically equivalent to the brand-name drug.

b. It designates a brand-name drug's price.

c. It denotes a controlled substance classification.

d. It indicates the expiration date of a medication.

75. In what circumstances can a pharmacist substitute a brand-name drug with a generic drug without consulting the prescriber?

a. Only when the patient requests a generic

b. Never; pharmacists must always consult the prescriber before making substitutions

c. When the generic drug has an AB rating in the Orange Book

d. Only when the prescriber is unavailable for consultation

76. What is the role of the "Therapeutic Equivalence Codes" in the Orange Book?

a. They indicate the drug's shelf life.

b. They provide pricing information for generic drugs.

c. They specify the drug's dosage form.

d. They help healthcare professionals identify therapeutically equivalent drug products.

77. Which federal law governs the substitution of generic drugs for brand-name drugs by pharmacists?

a. Federal Food, Drug, and Cosmetic Act (FDCA)

b. Drug Price Competition and Patent Term Restoration Act (Hatch-Waxman Act)

c. Drug Enforcement Administration (DEA) regulations

d. Controlled Substances Act (CSA)

78. Which federal agency is primarily responsible for regulating and overseeing opioid treatment programs (OTPs) in the United States?

a. Drug Enforcement Administration (DEA)

b. Food and Drug Administration (FDA)

c. Substance Abuse and Mental Health Services Administration (SAMHSA)

d. Centers for Disease Control and Prevention (CDC)

79. What is the primary medication used in opioid treatment programs to help individuals with opioid use disorder?

a. Methadone

b. Oxycodone

c. Fentanyl

d. Hydrocodone

80. What are the main components of medication-assisted treatment (MAT) in opioid treatment programs?

a. Medication, counseling, and psychosocial support

b. Medication only

c. Counseling and psychosocial support only

d. Counseling only

81. What federal law allows qualified healthcare providers to prescribe buprenorphine for the treatment of opioid use disorder outside of traditional OTPs?

a. Drug Addiction Treatment Act (DATA 2000)

b. Controlled Substances Act (CSA)

c. Drug Enforcement Administration (DEA) regulations

d. Ryan Haight Online Pharmacy Consumer Protection Act

82. How are patients typically assessed for admission to an opioid treatment program (OTP)?

   a. Patients must pass a drug test.

   b. Patients are evaluated based on their insurance coverage.

   c. Patients are assessed for opioid use disorder through clinical evaluation.

   d. Patients must complete a counseling program.

83. What is the purpose of DEA Form 222 in federal pharmacy law?

   a. To register a pharmacy with the Drug Enforcement Administration (DEA)

   b. To report theft or loss of controlled substances

   c. To order Schedule II controlled substances for legitimate medical or research purposes

   d. To request authorization for the disposal of expired medications

84. Which of the following statements about DEA Form 222 is correct?

   a. It can be used to order both Schedule II and Schedule III controlled substances.

   b. It is an electronic form that can be submitted online.

   c. It must be kept on file at the pharmacy for 30 days.

   d. It requires the signature of both the supplier and the purchaser.

85. How many copies of DEA Form 222 are typically involved in the ordering process?

a. One copy

b. Two copies

c. Three copies

d. Four copies

86. In the event of a theft or loss of completed DEA Form 222, what should the pharmacy do?

a. Report it to the FDA

b. Report it to the DEA immediately

c. Keep it on file for future reference

d. Submit a copy to the state pharmacy board

87. Which federal agency enforces compliance with the regulations surrounding DEA Form 222?

a. Food and Drug Administration (FDA)

b. Drug Enforcement Administration (DEA)

c. Centers for Disease Control and Prevention (CDC)

d. Federal Trade Commission (FTC)

88. What is the primary purpose of a prescription monitoring program (PMP) in federal pharmacy law?

a. To regulate the pricing of prescription drugs

b. To monitor and track the prescribing and dispensing of controlled substances

c. To approve the marketing and advertising of prescription drugs

d. To establish guidelines for compounding pharmacies

89. Which healthcare professionals are typically required to report controlled substance prescriptions to a PMP?

a. Only pharmacists

b. Only prescribers (physicians, nurse practitioners, etc.)

c. Both pharmacists and prescribers

d. Only law enforcement agencies

90. How frequently are healthcare professionals usually required to report prescription data to a PMP?

a. Monthly

b. Annually

c. Quarterly

d. Daily

91. What is the main goal of using a PMP in the context of patient care?

a. To identify patients who are likely to misuse prescription medications

b. To restrict access to controlled substances for all patients

c. To replace the need for drug testing in pain management

d. To track the use of over-the-counter medications

92. In federal pharmacy law, who typically has access to the information stored in a PMP database?

a. The general public

b. Only pharmacists and prescribers

c. Law enforcement agencies

d. Only the DEA

93. What is the primary objective of the Omnibus Budget Reconciliation Act (OBRA) of 1990 concerning federal pharmacy law?

a. To establish a national formulary for prescription medications

b. To regulate the pricing of over-the-counter (OTC) medications

c. To improve the quality of care in long-term care facilities through medication management

d. To restrict the use of generic medications in favor of brand-name drugs

94. What key requirement did OBRA 1990 impose on pharmacists in the context of federal pharmacy law?

a. Mandatory drug pricing disclosures to patients

b. Mandatory counseling for Medicaid patients on new prescription medications

c. Mandatory prescription compounding for Medicaid patients

d. Mandatory pharmaceutical advertising for generic medications

95. Which federal agency oversees the implementation of OBRA 1990 provisions related to Medicaid and prescription drug coverage?

a. Drug Enforcement Administration (DEA)

b. Food and Drug Administration (FDA)

c. Centers for Medicare & Medicaid Services (CMS)

d. Substance Abuse and Mental Health Services Administration (SAMHSA)

96. What is the primary goal of the Drug Utilization Review (DUR) program mandated by OBRA 1990?

a. To promote the use of brand-name drugs over generic equivalents

b. To limit Medicaid beneficiaries' access to certain prescription medications

c. To prevent medication errors and ensure appropriate drug therapy

d. To reduce the number of pharmacies participating in Medicaid programs

97. How did OBRA 1990 impact the reimbursement of prescription medications for Medicaid beneficiaries?

    a. It increased the cost-sharing requirements for beneficiaries.

    b. It established a single, uniform reimbursement rate for all pharmacies.

    c. It allowed for additional reimbursement to pharmacies for counseling services.

    d. It eliminated prescription drug coverage for Medicaid beneficiaries.

98. What is the primary purpose of the Health Insurance Portability and Accountability Act (HIPAA) in the context of federal pharmacy law?

    a. To regulate the pricing of prescription medications

    b. To protect the privacy and security of patients' health information

    c. To establish federal guidelines for pharmaceutical advertising

    d. To standardize prescription drug labeling

99. Under HIPAA, what type of information is considered protected health information (PHI)?

    a. Any information related to an individual's medical history

    b. Any information related to an individual's insurance coverage

    c. Any individually identifiable health information

    d. Any information provided by a healthcare professional

100. Which healthcare entity or provider is considered a covered entity under HIPAA and is subject to its privacy and security regulations?

a. Pharmacies only

b. Health insurance companies only

c. Healthcare providers, health plans, and healthcare clearinghouses

d. Patients and their families

6. FEDERAL PHARMACY LAW ANSWERS PART-6

1. **Answer: B**

   The manufacturer or distributor

   Explanation: The manufacturer or distributor of a pharmaceutical product has the primary responsibility for initiating a recall when safety concerns or product defects are identified.

2. **Answer: C**

   Food and Drug Administration (FDA)

   Explanation: The FDA is responsible for overseeing and enforcing pharmaceutical recalls to protect public health and safety.

3. **Answer: C**

   To address a defect that could cause serious harm or death

   Explanation: Class I recalls are initiated when there is a reasonable probability that the use of or exposure to a product will cause serious adverse health consequences or death.

4. **Answer: B**

   Quarantine the recalled product and stop dispensing it immediately

   Explanation: The most important initial action for a pharmacy is to quarantine the recalled product and stop dispensing it to prevent further distribution to patients.

5. **Answer: C**

Wait for the FDA to provide instructions before taking any action

Explanation: Pharmacies should not wait for FDA instructions but should take immediate action upon receiving a recall notice, including notifying patients, documenting actions, and returning the recalled product to the manufacturer or distributor when appropriate. Waiting for FDA instructions could delay necessary actions to protect patients' health.

6. **Answer: C**

Schedule III

Explanation: Schedule III controlled substances have a moderate to low potential for physical and psychological dependence compared to Schedule I and II substances.

7. **Answer: B**

Nurse practitioners and physician assistants

Explanation: Nurse practitioners and physician assistants, in addition to physicians, have the authority to prescribe Schedule III and IV controlled substances under federal law, subject to state regulations.

8. **Answer: C**

Five refills within 6 months

Explanation: Under federal law, Schedule III and IV controlled substance prescriptions can have up to five refills within a 6-month period.

9. **Answer: C**

30 days

Explanation: Federal law generally allows for a 30-day supply of Schedule III and IV controlled substances per prescription.

10. **Answer: A**

Drug Enforcement Administration (DEA)

Explanation: The DEA is responsible for enforcing regulations related to controlled substances, including Schedule III and IV drugs.

11. **Answer: C**

Hydrocodone (Vicodin)

Explanation: Hydrocodone is typically classified as a Schedule II controlled substance, not Schedule IV.

12. **Answer: A**

Its potential for abuse

Explanation: The potential for abuse is a primary factor in determining a controlled substance's schedule classification, with Schedule I having the highest potential for abuse and Schedule V having the lowest.

13. **Answer: A**

Schedule I

Explanation: Schedule I controlled substances have a high potential for abuse and no accepted medical use in the United States.

14. **Answer: C**

To regulate the manufacturing and distribution of controlled substances

Explanation: The primary purpose of scheduling controlled substances is to regulate their manufacturing, distribution, and use to prevent abuse and diversion.

15. **Answer: D**

Nurse practitioners, physician assistants, and pharmacists

Explanation: Nurse practitioners, physician assistants, and pharmacists, in addition to physicians, can dispense Schedule III and IV controlled substances to patients in accordance with federal and state regulations.

16. **Answer: B**

Twice

Explanation: Under federal law, a Schedule III to V prescription can be transferred between pharmacies only once. However, if it is not fully dispensed after the first transfer, it can be transferred one more time, totaling two transfers.

17. **Answer: D**

All of the above

Explanation: Under federal law, pharmacists, pharmacy technicians, nurse practitioners, physician assistants, and prescribing physicians can initiate the transfer of a Schedule III to V prescription, subject to state regulations.

18. **Answer: D**

National Provider Identifier (NPI) of the prescribing healthcare provider

Explanation: The NPI of the prescribing healthcare provider is not typically required on the prescription transfer record; instead, the name and DEA number of the prescriber are typically recorded.

19. **Answer: B**

14 days

Explanation: Federal law allows up to 14 days for completing the transfer of a Schedule III to V prescription, including the initial dispense by the receiving pharmacy.

20. **Answer: C**

Prescription number, patient's name, and the quantity dispensed

Explanation: When transferring a Schedule III to V prescription, federal law requires communication of the prescription number, patient's name, and the quantity dispensed to the receiving pharmacy.

21. **Answer: C**

Schedule III

Explanation: Medications with a moderate potential for abuse and accepted medical use are classified as Schedule III controlled substances.

22. **Answer: A**

The Controlled Substances Act (CSA)

Explanation: The transfer of Schedule III to V prescriptions between pharmacies is primarily governed by the Controlled Substances Act (CSA).

23. Answer: A

Drug Enforcement Administration (DEA)

Explanation: The DEA is responsible for enforcing the regulations related to controlled substances, including prescription transfers.

24. Answer: C

A 30-day supply

Explanation: The maximum allowable quantity of a Schedule III to V controlled substance that can be transferred between pharmacies is typically a 30-day supply.

25. Answer: B

18 years old

Explanation: Under federal law, pharmacy technicians involved in the transfer of Schedule III to V prescriptions must typically be at least 18 years old, although specific state requirements may vary.

26. Answer: A

Medicare

Explanation: Medicare is a federal program that primarily provides healthcare coverage for individuals aged 65 and older and some younger individuals with specific disabilities.

27. Answer: C

Centers for Medicare & Medicaid Services (CMS)

Explanation: CMS is the federal agency responsible for administering the Medicare program, including its prescription drug coverage, known as Medicare Part D.

28. **Answer: D**

Medicare Part D

Explanation: Medicare Part D is the part of Medicare that covers prescription drug benefits for Medicare beneficiaries.

29. **Answer: B**

Low-income individuals and families

Explanation: Medicaid is a joint federal and state program designed to provide healthcare coverage to low-income individuals and families.

30. **Answer: C**

Centers for Medicare & Medicaid Services (CMS)

Explanation: CMS is responsible for overseeing the Medicaid program at the federal level and establishing federal regulations and guidelines for the program.

31. **Answer: B**

Affordable Care Act (ACA)

Explanation: The Affordable Care Act (ACA) expanded Medicaid eligibility in participating states to include more low-income adults, increasing access to healthcare coverage.

32. **Answer: D**

Medicare Part D regulations

Explanation: Pharmacies that participate in Medicare Part D must adhere to the regulations specific to that program, including those related to prescription drug coverage and claims processing.

33. Answer: B

Age

Explanation: While age is a factor considered for Medicare eligibility, it is not a primary factor for Medicaid eligibility, which is primarily based on income, disability status, and citizenship or immigration status.

34. Answer: C

CHIP (Children's Health Insurance Program)

Explanation: CHIP is a federal program that provides healthcare coverage for low-income children in the United States, while Medicaid primarily serves low-income individuals and families.

35. Answer: C

To ensure the safe and effective use of prescription medications

Explanation: The Drug Utilization Review (DUR) program in Medicaid aims to ensure the safe and effective use of prescription medications by beneficiaries, rather than limiting access or increasing costs.

36. Answer: C

Drug Enforcement Administration (DEA)

Explanation: The DEA is the federal agency primarily responsible for regulating and enforcing laws related to controlled substances, ensuring their safe and legal use.

37. Answer: B

To reduce the availability of controlled substances

Explanation: The DEA's primary mission is to reduce the availability of controlled substances for illegal purposes while ensuring their availability for legitimate medical and scientific purposes.

38. Answer: C

Food and Drug Administration (FDA)

Explanation: The FDA is responsible for approving new drugs for marketing in the United States and overseeing their safety and efficacy throughout their lifecycle.

39. Answer: B

To evaluate and approve new drugs

Explanation: CDER within the FDA is responsible for evaluating and approving new drugs for marketing in the United States.

40. Answer: A

The FDA does not regulate dietary supplements.

Explanation: The FDA does not regulate dietary supplements in the same way it regulates prescription and over-the-counter drugs. Dietary supplements are regulated under the Dietary Supplement Health and Education Act (DSHEA).

41. Answer: B

Centers for Disease Control and Prevention (CDC)

Explanation: The CDC is responsible for tracking and investigating outbreaks of foodborne illnesses, while the FDA is primarily responsible for ensuring the safety of the food supply.

42. Answer: B

To oversee the safety of vaccines and blood products

Explanation: CBER within the FDA is responsible for regulating and ensuring the safety of vaccines, blood products, and related biologics.

43. Answer: B

Pharmacists

Explanation: The DEA assigns a unique registration number to pharmacists, allowing them to handle and dispense controlled substances.

44. Answer: B

To track adverse events and safety concerns related to medications and medical products

Explanation: The FDA's MedWatch program is designed to track and report adverse events and safety concerns related to medications and medical products.

45. Answer: C

Food and Drug Administration (FDA)

Explanation: The FDA is responsible for regulating the labeling and advertising of tobacco products under the Family Smoking Prevention and Tobacco Control Act.

46. Answer: C

FDA

Explanation: The Food and Drug Administration (FDA) is the primary federal agency responsible for regulating medication development, production, and marketing in the United States.

47. Answer: A

Drug Enforcement Administration

Explanation: The DEA, or Drug Enforcement Administration, plays a role in regulating controlled substances and enforcing drug-related laws.

48. Answer: B

Available without a prescription

Explanation: Over-the-counter (OTC) medications are available to consumers without a prescription, as opposed to prescription-only medications.

49. Answer: B

Generic drug approval

Explanation: The Hatch-Waxman Act is primarily related to the regulation and approval of generic drugs.

50. Answer: D

Risk management for certain medications

Explanation: REMS are strategies implemented by the FDA to manage and mitigate the risks associated with certain medications.

51. **Answer: C**

It enforces regulations to ensure accurate and balanced drug promotion.

Explanation: The FDA has authority over drug advertising and ensures that it is accurate and not misleading.

52. **Answer: B**

To encourage the development of medications for rare diseases

Explanation: The Orphan Drug Act provides incentives to pharmaceutical companies to develop medications for rare diseases.

53. **Answer: B**

Medication safety

Explanation: GMPs ensure that pharmaceutical products are consistently produced and controlled to meet quality standards and safety requirements.

54. **Answer: B**

Generic versions of biologic drugs

Explanation: Biosimilars are highly similar, but not identical, versions of biologic drugs.

55. **Answer: C**

It addresses tampering and contamination issues with OTC products.

Explanation: The Federal Anti-Tampering Act is designed to prevent tampering with consumer products, including OTC medications.

56. **Answer: B**

It enforces antitrust laws within the pharmaceutical industry.

Explanation: The FTC enforces competition and antitrust laws in various industries, including pharmaceuticals.

57. **Answer: C**

Enhancing medication safety and tracing

Explanation: The DSCSA aims to improve the security and traceability of the pharmaceutical supply chain.

58. **Answer: C**

Food and Drug Administration (FDA)

Explanation: The FDA is the primary federal agency responsible for regulating the approval, safety, and oversight of biologic drugs in the United States.

59. **Answer: C**

Biologics are typically derived from living organisms.

Explanation: Biologic drugs are typically large, complex molecules derived from living organisms or produced using biotechnology processes, while traditional small-molecule drugs are chemically synthesized.

60. **Answer: B**

Biologics License Application (BLA)

Explanation: Biosimilars are approved through the Biologics License Application (BLA) pathway, which is distinct from the pathway used for traditional small-molecule generic drugs (ANDA).

61. **Answer: B**

It lists approved biosimilar products.

Explanation: The Purple Book is a publication by the FDA that lists approved biologic products and their biosimilars, helping healthcare professionals and the public identify these products.

62. **Answer: B**

Promoting the development of biosimilars

Explanation: The BPCIA is a federal law that encourages the development and approval of biosimilars to increase competition and reduce the cost of biologic drugs.

63. **Answer: C**

Food and Drug Administration (FDA)

Explanation: The FDA is responsible for regulating and providing guidelines for prescription drug labeling information for the patient, ensuring it is accurate and informative.

64. **Answer: C**

Information on the drug's manufacturer

Explanation: The "Patient Information" section typically includes dosage instructions, potential side effects, and storage instructions, but it does not usually provide information on the drug's manufacturer.

65. Answer: B

To emphasize the potential for severe or life-threatening side effects

Explanation: A Black Box Warning is used to draw attention to serious or life-threatening risks associated with a medication.

66. Answer: B

It offers guidance on how to administer the drug to patients.

Explanation: The "Instructions for Use" section provides guidance on how patients should properly administer the medication, including any special instructions.

67. Answer: D

The Drug Facts panel

Explanation: The "Drug Facts" label is the standard format for presenting essential information on OTC medication packaging, required by the FDA to provide clear and concise information to consumers.

68. Answer: A

Compounding is performed by pharmacists, while manufacturing is done by pharmaceutical companies.

Explanation: The primary distinction is that compounding is the preparation of personalized medications by pharmacists or physicians for individual patients, while manufacturing is the large-scale production of commercial drug products by pharmaceutical companies.

69. **Answer: B**

Drug Quality and Security Act (DQSA)

Explanation: The Drug Quality and Security Act (DQSA) amended the FDCA to provide specific regulations and standards for pharmacy compounding.

70. **Answer: B**

USP provides guidance for pharmacy compounding practices.

Explanation: USP provides standards and guidance for the quality and safety of compounded medications, ensuring they meet specific requirements.

71. **Answer: A**

Outsourcing compounding facilities are subject to the same regulations as traditional pharmacies.

Explanation: Outsourcing compounding facilities must adhere to the same regulations and standards as traditional pharmacies to ensure the safety and quality of compounded medications.

72. **Answer: B**

When a compounding pharmacy uses bulk drug substances that are not on an FDA-approved list

Explanation: The FDA may exercise stricter regulatory oversight if a compounding pharmacy uses bulk drug substances that are not on an FDA-approved list or if other criteria are met, as outlined in the DQSA.

73. Answer: B

A publication listing generic drug products and their equivalence to brand-name drugs

Explanation: The Orange Book is a publication by the FDA that lists approved drug products, including generic drug products, and their therapeutic equivalence to brand-name drugs.

74. Answer: A

It signifies that a generic drug product is therapeutically equivalent to the brand-name drug.

Explanation: An AB rating in the Orange Book indicates that the generic drug product is considered therapeutically equivalent to the brand-name drug, allowing for substitution.

75. Answer: C

When the generic drug has an AB rating in the Orange Book

Explanation: Pharmacists can typically substitute a brand-name drug with a generic drug if the generic has an AB rating in the Orange Book, without the need for prescriber consultation.

76. Answer: D

They help healthcare professionals identify therapeutically equivalent drug products.

Explanation: Therapeutic Equivalence Codes in the Orange Book assist healthcare professionals in identifying drug products that are therapeutically equivalent to one another.

77. Answer: B

Drug Price Competition and Patent Term Restoration Act (Hatch-Waxman Act)

Explanation: The Hatch-Waxman Act establishes the legal framework for generic drug substitution by pharmacists in the United States.

78. Answer: C

Substance Abuse and Mental Health Services Administration (SAMHSA)

Explanation: SAMHSA is the federal agency responsible for regulating and overseeing OTPs to ensure the safe and effective treatment of opioid use disorder.

79. Answer: A

Methadone

Explanation: Methadone is a medication commonly used in opioid treatment programs to help individuals manage and overcome opioid addiction.

80. Answer: A

Medication, counseling, and psychosocial support

Explanation: MAT in opioid treatment programs typically includes medication, counseling, and psychosocial support to provide comprehensive treatment.

81. Answer: A

Drug Addiction Treatment Act (DATA 2000)

Explanation: DATA 2000 allows qualified healthcare providers to obtain a waiver to prescribe buprenorphine in office-based settings for opioid use disorder treatment.

82. Answer: C

Patients are assessed for opioid use disorder through clinical evaluation.

Explanation: Admission to an OTP usually involves a clinical evaluation to determine the presence and severity of opioid use disorder, which helps determine the appropriate treatment plan.

83. Answer: C

To order Schedule II controlled substances for legitimate medical or research purposes

Explanation: DEA Form 222 is used to order Schedule II controlled substances for legitimate medical or research purposes, serving as a record of the transaction.

84. Answer: D

It requires the signature of both the supplier and the purchaser.

Explanation: DEA Form 222 requires the signature of both the supplier (registrant) and the purchaser (pharmacy) to complete the order.

85. Answer: B

Two copies

Explanation: Typically, two copies of DEA Form 222 are involved in the ordering process: one is sent to the supplier, and the other is retained by the purchaser.

86. Answer: B

Report it to the DEA immediately

Explanation: In the event of a theft or loss of a completed DEA Form 222, the pharmacy should report it to the DEA immediately to prevent unauthorized orders.

87. Answer: B

Drug Enforcement Administration (DEA)

Explanation: The DEA is responsible for enforcing compliance with the regulations surrounding DEA Form 222 and controlled substance ordering.

88. Answer: B

To monitor and track the prescribing and dispensing of controlled substances

Explanation: The primary purpose of a PMP is to monitor and track the prescribing and dispensing of controlled substances to help prevent misuse and diversion.

89. Answer: C

Both pharmacists and prescribers

Explanation: Both pharmacists and prescribers are typically required to report controlled substance prescriptions to a PMP to ensure comprehensive tracking.

90. Answer: D

Daily

Explanation: In many jurisdictions, healthcare professionals are required to report prescription data to a PMP on a daily basis to provide up-to-date information.

91. Answer: A

To identify patients who are likely to misuse prescription medications

Explanation: One of the primary goals of a PMP is to identify patients who may be at risk of misusing or abusing prescription medications so that appropriate interventions can be implemented.

92. Answer: B

Only pharmacists and prescribers

Explanation: Generally, only pharmacists and prescribers with a legitimate need to access PMP data are granted access to the information for patient care purposes, not the general public.

93. Answer: C

To improve the quality of care in long-term care facilities through medication management

Explanation: OBRA 1990 included provisions to enhance the quality of care for residents in long-term care facilities, emphasizing medication management and the role of pharmacists.

94. Answer: B

Mandatory counseling for Medicaid patients on new prescription medications

Explanation: OBRA 1990 required pharmacists to offer counseling to Medicaid patients receiving new prescription medications to ensure they understood proper medication use.

95. Answer: C

Centers for Medicare & Medicaid Services (CMS)

Explanation: CMS oversees the implementation of OBRA 1990 provisions related to Medicaid and prescription drug coverage.

96. Answer: C

To prevent medication errors and ensure appropriate drug therapy

Explanation: The DUR program required states to establish procedures for prospective and retrospective drug use reviews to prevent medication errors and ensure appropriate drug therapy.

97. Answer: C

It allowed for additional reimbursement to pharmacies for counseling services.

Explanation: OBRA 1990 provided for additional reimbursement to pharmacies for the provision of counseling services to Medicaid beneficiaries, incentivizing pharmacists to offer counseling as required.

98. Answer: B

To protect the privacy and security of patients' health information

Explanation: HIPAA's primary purpose is to safeguard the privacy and security of patients' protected health information (PHI), including their medical and prescription records.

99. Answer: C

Any individually identifiable health information

Explanation: PHI includes any individually identifiable health information, such as medical records, prescriptions, and billing information.

100. Answer: C

Healthcare providers, health plans, and healthcare clearinghouses

Explanation: Covered entities under HIPAA include healthcare providers, health plans, and healthcare clearinghouses, which may encompass pharmacies, hospitals, insurance companies, and more.

7. FEDERAL PHARMACY LAW QUESTIONS PART-7

1. Which of the following is an example of a commonly abused prescription opioid?

   a. Ibuprofen

   b. Acetaminophen

   c. Oxycodone

   d. Naproxen

2. Which of the following is not a common sign of opioid overdose?

   a. Pinpoint pupils

   b. Slow or shallow breathing

   c. Increased heart rate

   d. Loss of consciousness

3. Which of the following is not a common side effect of benzodiazepines?

   a. Dizziness

   b. Memory loss

   c. Increased energy

   d. Sedation

4. . Which of the following is not a common method of illicitly obtaining prescription drugs?

   a. Doctor shopping

   b. Prescription forgery

   c. Online pharmacies

   d. Properly obtaining a prescription from a healthcare provider

5. . Which of the following is not a common treatment option for opioid use disorder?

   a. Methadone maintenance therapy

   b. Cognitive-behavioral therapy

   c. Naltrexone (Vivitrol) injections

   d. Increasing the dosage of opioids

6. . Which of the following is not a common sign of stimulant abuse?

   a. Increased energy and alertness

   b. Weight loss

   c. Agitation and irritability

   d. Slurred speech

7. . Which of the following is not a common side effect of long-term steroid use?

    a. Increased muscle mass

    b. Mood swings

    c. Osteoporosis

    d. Increased risk of infection

8. Which of the following is not a common hallucinogenic substance?

    a. LSD

    b. Psilocybin (magic mushrooms)

    c. MDMA (ecstasy)

    d. Methamphetamine

9. Which of the following is not a common sign of marijuana use?

    a. Bloodshot eyes

    b. Increased appetite

    c. Slowed reaction time

    d. Decreased heart rate

10. Which of the following is not a common sign of sedative-hypnotic use?

    a. Drowsiness

    b. Slurred speech

    c. Memory loss

    d. Increased heart rate

11. . Which of the following is not a common sign of hallucinogen use?

    a. Visual hallucinations

    b. Distorted perception of time

    c. Increased heart rate

    d. Altered sense of self

12. Which of the following is not a common side effect of long-term alcohol abuse?

    a. Liver damage

    b. Memory loss

    c. Increased risk of cancer

    d. Improved cognitive function

13. Which of the following is not a common sign of inhalant abuse?

    a. Slurred speech

    b. Dizziness

    c. Impaired coordination

    d. Nosebleeds

14. Which of the following is not a common sign of anabolic steroid abuse?

    a. Increased muscle mass

    b. Acne

    c. Mood swings

    d. Decreased libido

15. Which of the following is not a common treatment option for alcohol use disorder?

    a. Medications like naltrexone and acamprosate

    b. Support groups like Alcoholics Anonymous

    c. Detoxification programs

    d. Increasing alcohol consumption

16. Which of the following is not a common sign of synthetic cannabinoid use?

    a. Elevated mood

    b. Paranoia and anxiety

    c. Increased appetite

    d. Hallucinations

17. Which of the following is not a common side effect of long-term cocaine use?

    a. Increased risk of heart attack

    b. Nasal damage

    c. Weight gain

    d. Psychosis

18. Which of the following is not a common sign of club drug use?

    a. Euphoria

    b. Increased sociability

    c. Memory loss

    d. Decreased heart rate

19. Which of the following is not a common side effect of long-term methamphetamine use?

    a. Dental problems

    b. Skin sores

    c. Increased energy and focus

    d. Weight loss

20. Which of the following is not a common sign of prescription stimulant abuse?

    a. Increased alertness and focus

    b. Weight loss

    c. Agitation and irritability

    d. Slowed heart rate

21. Which federal agency is responsible for enforcing laws related to controlled substances in the United States?

    a. Drug Enforcement Administration (DEA)

    b. Food and Drug Administration (FDA)

    c. Centers for Disease Control and Prevention (CDC)

    d. Federal Bureau of Investigation (FBI)

22. Which schedule of controlled substances has the highest potential for abuse and no accepted medical use?

    a. Schedule I

    b. Schedule II

    c. Schedule III

    d. Schedule IV

23. Which of the following is not a requirement for a substance to be classified as a Schedule I controlled substance?

    a. High potential for abuse

    b. No currently accepted medical use

    c. Lack of safety for use under medical supervision

    d. Moderate potential for abuse and physical dependence

24. Which of the following is not a common penalty for illegal possession of a controlled substance?

    a. Fines

    b. Probation

    c. Community service

    d. Public apology

25. Which of the following is not a common penalty for illegal distribution of a controlled substance?

    a. Imprisonment

    b. Fines

    c. Loss of professional license

    d. Mandatory drug rehabilitation

26. Which of the following is not a common requirement for obtaining a prescription for a controlled substance?

    a. A valid medical condition

    b. A physical examination by a healthcare provider

    c. A written prescription from a licensed healthcare provider

    d. A valid driver's license

27. Which of the following is not a common restriction for prescribing controlled substances?

    a. Limiting the quantity of medication prescribed

    b. Requiring frequent follow-up appointments

    c. Requiring a second opinion from another healthcare provider

    d. Allowing patients to self-prescribe

28. Which of the following is not a common method of disposing of unused or expired controlled substances?

    a. Flushing them down the toilet

    b. Returning them to a pharmacy or law enforcement agency

    c. Mixing them with undesirable substances (e.g., coffee grounds) and throwing them in the trash

    d. Participating in a drug take-back program

29. Which of the following is not a common requirement for operating a pharmacy that dispenses controlled substances?

    a. Obtaining a valid license from the state pharmacy board

    b. Maintaining accurate records of controlled substance transactions

    c. Conducting regular inventory checks of controlled substances

    d. Allowing customers to purchase controlled substances without a prescription

30. Which of the following is not a common restriction for advertising controlled substances?

    a. Prohibiting false or misleading claims

    b. Requiring disclosure of potential side effects and risks

    c. Allowing direct-to-consumer advertising for Schedule II substances

    d. Ensuring advertisements are approved by regulatory authorities

31. Which federal agency is responsible for regulating controlled substances in the United States?

    a. FDA (Food and Drug Administration)

    b. DEA (Drug Enforcement Administration)

    c. CDC (Centers for Disease Control and Prevention)

    d. NIH (National Institutes of Health)

32. Which schedule of controlled substances has the highest potential for abuse and no accepted medical use?

    a. Schedule I

    b. Schedule II

    c. Schedule III

    d. Schedule IV

33. Which of the following is an example of a Schedule II controlled substance?

    a. Codeine

    b. Xanax

    c. Vicodin

    d. Marijuana

34. How often must a pharmacy conduct an inventory of controlled substances?

    a. Monthly

    b. Quarterly

    c. Annually

    d. Biennially

35. Which of the following is not a requirement for prescribing Schedule II controlled substances?

    a. A written prescription with the prescriber's signature

    b. A DEA registration number on the prescription

    c. A maximum of five refills within six months

    d. A valid medical purpose

36. Which of the following is an example of a Schedule III controlled substance?

    a. Oxycodone

    b. Adderall

    c. Ketamine

    d. Ambien

37. Which schedule of controlled substances has the lowest potential for abuse and accepted medical use?

    a. Schedule I

    b. Schedule II

    c. Schedule III

    d. Schedule V

38. Which of the following is not a requirement for dispensing controlled substances?

    a. Verifying the patient's identity

    b. Recording the patient's address

    c. Documenting the quantity dispensed

    d. Obtaining the patient's social security number

39. Which of the following is an example of a Schedule IV controlled substance?

    a. Heroin

    b. LSD

    c. Valium

    d. Methamphetamine

40. Which of the following is not a factor considered when determining the schedule of a controlled substance?

    a. Potential for abuse

    b. Accepted medical use

    c. Cost of production

    d. Safety profile

41. Which of the following is an example of a Schedule V controlled substance?

    a. Fentanyl

    b. Cocaine

    c. Lysergic acid diethylamide (LSD)

    d. Cough syrup with codeine

42. Which of the following is not a requirement for storing controlled substances securely?

    a. Keeping them in a locked cabinet or safe

    b. Limiting access to authorized personnel only

    c. Maintaining a log of all controlled substance transactions

    d. Storing them in a visible and easily accessible area

43. Which of the following is not a common side effect of opioid analgesics?

    a. Constipation

    b. Drowsiness

    c. Increased heart rate

    d. Respiratory depression

44. Which of the following is not a valid reason for a prescriber to prescribe a controlled substance?

    a. To treat severe pain

    b. To manage anxiety or insomnia

    c. To induce euphoria or recreational use

    d. To alleviate symptoms of attention deficit hyperactivity disorder (ADHD)

45. Which of the following is not a requirement for documenting controlled substance dispensing?

    a. Date of dispensing

    b. Patient's age and gender

    c. Quantity dispensed

    d. Prescriber's DEA registration number

46. Which of the following is an example of a Schedule II stimulant?

    a. Ritalin

    b. Xanax

    c. Ambien

    d. Ativan

47. Which of the following is not a requirement for reporting controlled substance prescriptions to a prescription drug monitoring program (PDMP)?

    a. Reporting within 24-72 hours of dispensing

    b. Reporting patient information such as name and address

    c. Reporting the quantity and strength of the controlled substance

    d. Reporting the patient's social security number

48. Which of the following is not a factor that contributes to the opioid crisis?

    a. Overprescribing of opioids

    b. Illicit drug trafficking

    c. Lack of access to addiction treatment

    d. Strict regulations on controlled substances

49. Which of the following is not a valid method for disposing of unused or expired controlled substances?

    a. Flushing them down the toilet

    b. Returning them to a DEA-authorized collector

    c. Participating in a drug take-back program

    d. Mixing them with undesirable substances (e.g., coffee grounds) and throwing them in the trash

50. Which of the following is not a requirement for prescribing controlled substances via telemedicine?

    a. The patient must be physically located in a healthcare facility

    b. The prescriber must comply with state and federal regulations

    c. The prescriber must establish a valid patient-prescriber relationship

    d. The prescriber must conduct a thorough medical evaluation

51. Why does the government heavily regulate medicinal drugs?

    a. To restrict individual choices

    b. To protect people from potential risks

    c. To promote risky behavior

    d. To encourage self-medication

52. Which of the following is NOT a relevant market failure related to drug use?

    a. Public goods

    b. Externalities

    c. Natural monopolies

    d. Information asymmetry

53. Why is government interference with private choices to use medicinal drugs justified?

    a. To promote risky behavior

    b. To restrict individual choices

    c. To address market failures

    d. To encourage self-medication

54. Why is the regulation of vaccines necessary?

    a. To restrict individual choices

    b. To promote risky behavior

    c. To prevent epidemics and protect society

    d. To encourage self-medication

55. Why are vaccines viewed as too risky by many individuals?

    a. Because they have no benefit to the individual

    b. Because they have no benefit to society

    c. Because of acute reactions to them

    d. Because they are expensive

56. Why is government regulation required for vaccinations?

    a. To restrict individual choices

    b. To promote risky behavior

    c. To prevent epidemics and protect society

    d. To encourage self-medication

57. What is a public good related to vaccines?

    a. Individual benefit

    b. Prevention of epidemics

    c. Acute reactions

    d. Mass product liability actions

58. Why did most manufacturers stop producing childhood vaccines?

   a. Because of government regulations

   b. Because of public goods

   c. Because of externalities

   d. Because of mass product liability actions

59. What is the benefit of vaccines to society as a whole?

   a. Individual benefit

   b. Prevention of epidemics

   c. Acute reactions

   d. Mass product liability actions

60. Why must the government ensure the availability of vaccines?

   a. To restrict individual choices

   b. To promote risky behavior

   c. To prevent epidemics and protect society

   d. To encourage self-medication

61. Which of the following is a regulated seller of SLCPs?

    a. A hospital

    b. A grocery store

    c. A manufacturing plant

    d. A research laboratory

62. Which of the following substances is not considered an SLCP?

    a. Ephedrine

    b. Pseudoephedrine

    c. Acetaminophen

    d. Phenylpropanolamine

63. What is the definition of a regulated seller?

    a. An employee or agent of a retail distributor

    b. A pharmacy engaged in the distribution of bulk quantities of SLCPs

    c. An entity engaged in over-the-counter sales of SLCPs directly to walk-in customers

    d. None of the above

64. What is the penalty for materially falsifying a DEA registration application?

    a. A warning letter

    b. A fine

    c. Suspension or revocation of registration

    d. None of the above

65. Which of the following can result in the suspension or revocation of a DEA registration?

    a. Conviction of a felony relating to a controlled substance or List I chemical

    b. Suspension, revocation, or denial of a state license or registration

    c. Materially falsifying a registration application

    d. All of the above

66. What is the requirement for a pharmacy that wants to distribute bulk quantities of SLCPs?

    a. Register with DEA as a chemical distributor

    b. Register as a regulated seller

    c. Obtain a state license

    d. None of the above

67. Which of the following is an example of a regulated seller?

    a. A research laboratory

    b. A hospital pharmacy

    c. A drug store

    d. A manufacturing plant

68. Which of the following substances can be classified as an SLCP?

    a. Acetaminophen

    b. Aspirin

    c. Ephedrine

    d. Ibuprofen

69. What is the penalty for having a state license or registration suspended, revoked, or denied by a competent state authority?

    a. A warning letter

    b. A fine

    c. Suspension or revocation of DEA registration

    d. None of the above

70. What is the penalty for selling SLCPs without a DEA registration?

    a. A warning letter

    b. A fine

    c. Suspension or revocation of DEA registration

    d. None of the above

71. Which of the following is not a requirement for a regulated seller?

    a. Registration with DEA

    b. Recordkeeping of SLCP sales

    c. Employee drug testing

    d. Compliance with state and federal laws

72. Which of the following is not an SLCP?

    a. Pseudoephedrine

    b. Phenylpropanolamine

    c. Methamphetamine

    d. Acetaminophen

73. What is the penalty for distributing SLCPs without proper recordkeeping?

   a. A warning letter

   b. A fine

   c. Suspension or revocation of DEA registration

   d. None of the above

74. Which of the following is required for a pharmacy engaged in the distribution of bulk quantities of SLCPs?

   a. Registration with DEA as a chemical distributor

   b. Registration as a regulated seller

   c. Compliance with state and federal laws

   d. All of the above

75. What is the penalty for distributing SLCPs to an unauthorized person?

   a. A warning letter

   b. A fine

   c. Suspension or revocation of DEA registration

   d. None of the above

76. Which of the following is not a List I chemical?

    a. Ephedrine

    b. Pseudoephedrine

    c. Acetaminophen

    d. Phenylpropanolamine

77. What is the penalty for distributing SLCPs in violation of state or federal law?

    a. A warning letters

    b. A fine

    c. Suspension or revocation of DEA registration

    d. None of the above

78. Which of the following is not a requirement for a chemical distributor?

    a. Registration with DEA

    b. Recordkeeping of chemical sales

    c. Compliance with state and federal laws

    d. Employee drug testing

79. What is the penalty for distributing SLCPs to a person who has exceeded the daily limit?

    a. A warning letters

    b. A fine

    c. Suspension or revocation of DEA registration

    d. None of the above

80. Which of the following is required for a pharmacy engaged in the distribution of bulk quantities of SLCPs?

    a. Registration with DEA as a regulated seller

    b. Registration with DEA as a chemical distributor

    c. Compliance with state and federal laws

    d. All of the above

81. What is the purpose of the DEA's Controlled Substance Ordering System (CSOS)?

    a. To restrict the ordering of schedule II-controlled substances

    b. To maintain records of electronic orders for controlled substances

    c. To promote the use of paper-based order forms

    d. To regulate the distribution of schedule II-controlled substances

82. Which entities are permitted to order schedule II-controlled substances electronically?

    a. Only pharmacies
    b. Only controlled substance manufacturers
    c. Only DEA authorized entities
    d. Only distributors

83. What technology does CSOS use for electronic ordering?

    a. Public Key Infrastructure (PKI)
    b. Digital certificates
    c. Certification Authority (CA)
    d. Electronic signatures

84. What is required for CSOS users to engage in electronic ordering?

    a. A digital signature issued by the DEA
    b. A digital certificate issued by the DEA
    c. A physical signature on paper-based order forms
    d. A certification from a DEA authorized entity

85. What is the role of the Certification Authority (CA) in CSOS?

    a. To restrict the use of electronic ordering

    b. To issue digital signatures for CSOS users

    c. To regulate the distribution of controlled substances

    d. To maintain records of electronic orders

86. When must a drug be inventoried as a controlled substance?

    a. When it is scheduled by the DEA

    b. When it is possessed by a registrant

    c. When it is ordered electronically

    d. When it is listed as a schedule II controlled substance

87. What is the effective date for inventorying a newly scheduled controlled substance?

    a. The date of electronic ordering

    b. The date of possession by a registrant

    c. The date of scheduling by the DEA

    d. The date of issuance of a digital certificate

88. What is the purpose of maintaining records of electronic orders?

    a. To restrict the use of controlled substances

    b. To track the distribution of controlled substances

    c. To promote the use of paper-based order forms

    d. To regulate the possession of controlled substances

89. What is the only electronic means of ordering schedule II controlled substances?

    a. CSOS

    b. PKI

    c. CA

    d. DEA authorized entities

90. Who is responsible for running the Certification Authority (CA) for CSOS?

    a. Controlled substance manufacturers

    b. Distributors

    c. Pharmacies

    d. DEA

91. Why must pharmacies maintain complete and accurate records for controlled substances?

    a. To restrict the dispensing of controlled substances

    b. To provide accountability for controlled substances

    c. To promote the diversion of controlled substances

    d. To reduce the manufacturing process of controlled substances

92. What is the purpose of the closed system for controlled substances?

    a. To increase the potential for diversion

    b. To restrict the accountability of controlled substances

    c. To promote the manufacturing process of controlled substances

    d. To reduce the potential for diversion

93. How many options do pharmacies have for filing paper prescription records?

    a. One option

    b. Two options

    c. Three options

    d. No options

94. Where should paper prescriptions for schedule II controlled substances be maintained?

   a. In a separate prescription file

   b. With the dispensing pharmacy

   c. At the registered location

   d. In the manufacturing process

95. What do federal requirements for filling prescriptions authorize or permit?

   a. Any act authorized by other federal laws

   b. Any act permitted by international treaties

   c. Any act permitted by state laws

   d. Any act authorized by the dispensing pharmacy

96. What should compliance with federal requirements for filling prescriptions be construed as?

   a. Compliance with other federal laws

   b. Compliance with state laws

   c. Compliance with international treaties

   d. Compliance with other federal or state laws unless expressly provided

97. What is the purpose of maintaining records for controlled substances?

    a. To restrict the dispensing of controlled substances

    b. To provide accountability for controlled substances

    c. To promote the diversion of controlled substances

    d. To increase the manufacturing process of controlled substances

98. What is the ultimate goal of the closed system for controlled substances?

    a. To increase the potential for diversion

    b. To restrict the accountability of controlled substances

    c. To promote the manufacturing process of controlled substances

    d. To reduce the potential for diversion

99. How should paper prescriptions for schedule II controlled substances be filed?

    a. In a separate prescription file

    b. With the dispensing pharmacy

    c. At the registered location

    d. In the manufacturing process

100.What should compliance with federal requirements for filling prescriptions not be construed as?

a. Compliance with other federal laws

b. Compliance with state laws

c. Compliance with international treaties

d. Compliance with the law of the state

7. FEDERAL PHARMACY LAW ANSWER PART-7

1. **Answer C**

   Oxycodone

2. **Answer C**

   Increased heart rate

3. **Answer C**

   Increased energy

4. **Answer D**

   Properly obtaining a prescription from a healthcare provider

5. **Answer D**

   Increasing the dosage of opioids

6. **Answer D**

   Slurred speech

7. **Answer A**

   Increased muscle mass

8. **Answer D**

   Methamphetamine

9. **Answer D**

Decreased heart rate

10. **Answer D**

Increased heart rate

11. **Answer C**

Increased heart rate

12. **Answer D**

Improved cognitive function

13. **Answer D**

Nosebleeds

14. **Answer. D**

Decreased libido

15. **Answer D**

Increasing alcohol consumption

16. **Answer C**

Increased appetite

17. **Answer C**

Weight gain

18. Answer D

Decreased heart rate

19. Answer C

Increased energy and focus

20. Answer D

Slowed heart rate

21. Answer A

Drug Enforcement Administration (DEA)

22. Answer A

Schedule I

23. Answer D

Moderate potential for abuse and physical dependence

24. Answer D

Public apology

25. Answer D

Mandatory drug rehabilitation

26. Answer D

A valid driver's license

27. Answer D

Allowing patients to self-prescribe

28. Answer A

Flushing them down the toilet

29. Answer D

Allowing customers to purchase controlled substances without a prescription

30. Answer C

Allowing direct-to-consumer advertising for Schedule II substances

31. Answer B

DEA (Drug Enforcement Administration)

32. Answer A

Schedule I

33. Answer D

Marijuana

34. Answer. C

Annually

35. Answer C

A maximum of five refills within six months

36. Answer C

Ketamine

37. Answer D

Schedule V

38. Answer D

Obtaining the patient's social security number

39. Answer C

Valium

40. Answer C

Cost of production

41. Answer D

Cough syrup with codeine

42. Answer D

Storing them in a visible and easily accessible area

43. Answer C

Increased heart rate

44. Answer C

To induce euphoria or recreational use

45. Answer D

Patient's age and gender

46. Answer A

Ritalin

47. Answer D

Reporting the patient's social security number

48. Answer D

Strict regulations on controlled substances

49. Answer A

Flushing them down the toilet

50. Answer A

The patient must be physically located in a healthcare facility

51. Answer B

To protect people from potential risks

52. Answer D

Information asymmetry

53. Answer C

To address market failures

54. Answer C

To prevent epidemics and protect society

55. Answer C

Because of acute reactions to them

56. Answer C

To prevent epidemics and protect society

57. Answer B

Prevention of epidemics

58. Answer D

Because of mass product liability actions

59. Answer B

Prevention of epidemics

60. Answer C

To prevent epidemics and protect society

61. Answer C

A manufacturing plant

62. Answer C

Acetaminophen

63. Answer C

An entity engaged in over-the-counter sales of SLCPs directly to walk-in customers

64. Answer C

Suspension or revocation of registration

65. Answer D

All of the above

66. Answer A

Register with DEA as a chemical distributor

67. Answer C

A drug store

68. Answer C

Ephedrine

69. Answer C

Suspension or revocation of DEA registration

70. Answer C

Suspension or revocation of DEA registration

71. Answer C

Employee drug testing

72. Answer D

Acetaminophen

73. Answer B

A fine

74. Answer D

All of the above

75. Answer C

Suspension or revocation of DEA registration

76. Answer C

Acetaminophen

77. Answer C

Suspension or revocation of DEA registration

78. Answer D

Employee drug testing

79. Answer B

A fine

80. Answer D

All of the above

81. Answer B

To maintain records of electronic orders for controlled substances

82. Answer C

Only DEA authorized entities

83. Answer A

Public Key Infrastructure (PKI)

84. Answer B

A digital certificate issued by the DEA

85. Answer B

To issue digital signatures for CSOS users

86. Answer A

When it is scheduled by the DEA

87. Answer C

The date of scheduling by the DEA

88. Answer B

To track the distribution of controlled substances

89. Answer A

CSOS

90. Answer D

DEA

91. Answer B

To provide accountability for controlled substances

92. Answer D

To reduce the potential for diversion

93. Answer B

Two options

94. Answer A

In a separate prescription file

95. Answer D

Any act authorized by other federal laws or permitted by international treaties, conventions, or protocols, or under the law of the state

96. Answer D

Compliance with other federal or state laws unless expressly provided

97. Answer B

To provide accountability for controlled substances

98. Answer D

To reduce the potential for diversion

99. Answer A

In a separate prescription file

100. Answer D

Compliance with the law of the state

8. FEDERAL PHARMACY LAW QUESTIONS PART-8

1. Which of the following is an example of a Schedule II controlled substance?

   a. Marijuana

   b. Heroin

   c. Xanax

   d. Codeine

2. Which federal agency is responsible for regulating the manufacturing and distribution of controlled substances?

   a. Drug Enforcement Administration (DEA)

   b. Food and Drug Administration (FDA)

   c. Centers for Disease Control and Prevention (CDC)

   d. National Institutes of Health (NIH)

3. Which of the following is not a common side effect of opioid use?

   a. Constipation

   b. Drowsiness

   c. Increased heart rate

   d. Respiratory depression

4. Which of the following is not a common sign of opioid withdrawal?

   a. Nausea and vomiting

   b. Muscle aches

   c. Dilated pupils

   d. Insomnia

5. Which of the following is not a common treatment option for opioid use disorder?

   a. Methadone maintenance therapy

   b. Cognitive-behavioral therapy

   c. Acupuncture

   d. Detoxification programs

6. Which of the following is not a common sign of benzodiazepine use?

   a. Sedation

   b. Memory impairment

   c. Increased energy

   d. Muscle relaxation

7. Which of the following is not a common side effect of long-term marijuana use?

   a. Impaired memory and concentration

   b. Increased appetite

   c. Lung damage

   d. Hallucinations

8. Which of the following is not a common sign of stimulant use?

   a. Increased energy and alertness

   b. Decreased appetite

   c. Paranoia and anxiety

   d. Slowed heart rate

9. Which of the following is not a common side effect of long-term hallucinogen use?

   a. Flashbacks

   b. Psychosis

   c. Increased creativity

   d. Mood swings

10. Which of the following is not a common sign of inhalant abuse?

    a. Slurred speech

    b. Dizziness

    c. Impaired coordination

    d. Increased heart rate

11. Which of the following is not a common sign of alcohol intoxication?

    a. Slurred speech

    b. Impaired coordination

    c. Increased heart rate

    d. Memory loss

12. Which of the following is not a common side effect of long-term alcohol abuse?

    a. Liver damage

    b. Cognitive impairment

    c. Increased risk of cancer

    d. Improved cardiovascular health

13. Which of the following is not a common sign of cocaine use?

    a. Euphoria

    b. Increased energy and alertness

    c. Dilated pupils

    d. Decreased heart rate

14. Which of the following is not a common side effect of long-term cocaine use?

    a. Paranoia and anxiety

    b. Respiratory problems

    c. Heart disease

    d. Weight loss

15. Which of the following is not a common sign of hallucinogen use?

    a. Altered perception of time and space

    b. Visual hallucinations

    c. Increased sociability

    d. Distorted sense of reality

16. Which of the following is not a common side effect of long-term hallucinogen use?

    a. Flashbacks

    b. Depression

    c. Increased empathy

    d. Memory problems

17. Which of the following is not a common sign of inhalant abuse?

    a. Slurred speech

    b. Nausea and vomiting

    c. Impaired judgment

    d. Red eyes

18. Which of the following is not a common side effect of long-term inhalant abuse?

    a. Liver damage

    b. Kidney damage

    c. Brain damage

    d. Peripheral neuropathy

19. Which of the following is not a common sign of prescription drug misuse?

    a. Increased tolerance

    b. Withdrawal symptoms

    c. Doctor shopping

    d. Improved sleep quality

20. Which of the following is not a common side effect of long-term prescription drug misuse?

    a. Addiction

    b. Organ damage

    c. Improved mental health

    d. Overdose

21. Which of the following is not a common sign of methamphetamine use?

    a. Increased energy and alertness

    b. Dilated pupils

    c. Weight loss

    d. Slowed heart rate

22. Which of the following is not a common side effect of long-term methamphetamine use?

    a. Dental problems

    b. Psychosis

    c. Memory loss

    d. Improved lung function

23. Which of the following is not a common sign of ecstasy (MDMA) use?

    a. Euphoria

    b. Increased empathy

    c. Increased body temperature

    d. Decreased blood pressure

24. Which of the following is not a common side effect of long-term ecstasy (MDMA) use?

    a. Depression

    b. Memory problems

    c. Liver damage

    d. Impaired immune function

25. Which of the following is not a common sign of anabolic steroid use?

    a. Increased muscle mass

    b. Acne

    c. Aggression and irritability

    d. Decreased libido

26. Which of the following is not a common side effect of long-term anabolic steroid use?

    a. Liver damage

    b. Cardiovascular problems

    c. Infertility

    d. Improved bone density

27. Which of the following is not a common sign of synthetic drug use (e.g., synthetic cannabinoids, bath salts)?

    a. Hallucinations

    b. Agitation and paranoia

    c. Increased appetite

    d. Seizures

28. Which of the following is not a common side effect of long-term synthetic drug use (e.g., synthetic cannabinoids, bath salts)?

    a. Kidney damage

    b. Psychosis

    c. Respiratory problems

    d. Improved cognitive function

29. Which of the following is not a common sign of inhalant abuse?

    a. Slurred speech

    b. Nausea and vomiting

    c. Impaired judgment

    d. Red eyes

30. Which of the following is not a common side effect of long-term inhalant abuse?

    a. Liver damage

    b. Kidney damage

    c. Brain damage

    d. Peripheral neuropathy

31. Which federal agency is responsible for enforcing laws related to controlled substances in the United States?

    a. Drug Enforcement Administration (DEA)

    b. Food and Drug Administration (FDA)

    c. Federal Bureau of Investigation (FBI)

    d. Central Intelligence Agency (CIA)

32. Which schedule of controlled substances includes drugs with the highest potential for abuse and no accepted medical use?

    a. Schedule I

    b. Schedule II

    c. Schedule III

    d. Schedule IV

33. Which of the following is not a requirement for a substance to be classified as a Schedule I controlled substance?

    a. High potential for abuse

    b. Accepted medical use

    c. Lack of accepted safety for use

    d. Lack of accepted safety for use under medical supervision

34. Which federal law regulates the manufacturing, distribution, and dispensing of controlled substances in the United States?

    a. Controlled Substances Act (CSA)

    b. Food, Drug, and Cosmetic Act (FDCA)

    c. Drug Enforcement Act (DEA)

    d. Substance Abuse and Mental Health Services Act (SAMHSA)

35. Which of the following is not a common penalty for the illegal possession of a controlled substance?

    a. Fines

    b. Probation

    c. Community service

    d. Public apology

36. Which of the following is not a common penalty for the illegal sale or distribution of a controlled substance?

    a. Imprisonment

    b. Fines

    c. Loss of professional license

    d. Mandatory drug rehabilitation

37. Which of the following is not a common penalty for the illegal manufacturing of a controlled substance?

    a. Imprisonment

    b. Fines

    c. Seizure of assets

    d. Public warning

38. Which of the following is not a common penalty for the illegal trafficking of a controlled substance?

    a. Imprisonment

    b. Fines

    c. Asset forfeiture

    d. Community service

39. Which of the following is not a common penalty for the illegal possession of drug paraphernalia?

    a. Fines

    b. Probation

    c. Mandatory drug testing

    d. Community service

40. Which of the following is not a common penalty for driving under the influence of a controlled substance?

    a. License suspension

    b. Fines

    c. Mandatory drug education programs

    d. Increased insurance premiums

41. Which federal agency has granted exceptions to the facsimile prescription requirements for Schedule II controlled substances?

    a. FDA

    b. DEA

    c. CDC

    d. NIH

42. Under what circumstances can a facsimile of a Schedule II prescription serve as the original prescription?

    a. When the prescription is for a compounded medication

    b. When the prescription is for a controlled substance administered parenterally

    c. When the prescription is for a controlled substance administered intravenously

    d. All of the above

43. What are the acceptable methods of administration for a compounded Schedule II narcotic controlled substance?

    a. Parenteral

    b. Intravenous

    c. Intramuscular

    d. All of the above

44. What type of facilities are eligible for the exception allowing facsimile transmission of Schedule II prescriptions?

    a. Hospitals

    b. Long-Term Care Facilities

    c. Rehabilitation centers

    d. All healthcare facilities

45. Who can transmit a prescription for Schedule II controlled substances to the dispensing pharmacy on behalf of a practitioner?

    a. The practitioner's assistant

    b. The practitioner's nurse

    c. The practitioner's authorized agent

    d. All of the above

46. How many exceptions have been granted by the DEA for facsimile prescriptions of Schedule II controlled substances?

    a. One

    b. Two

    c. Three

    d. Four

47. What is the purpose of the exceptions for facsimile prescriptions of Schedule II controlled substances?

    a. To simplify the prescription process for healthcare providers

    b. To ensure timely access to necessary medications for patients

    c. To reduce the risk of prescription errors

    d. All of the above

48. What is the maximum number of refills allowed for a Schedule II controlled substance prescription?

    a. No refills are allowed

    b. One refill is allowed

    c. Two refills are allowed

    d. Three refills are allowed

49. What documentation is required when a facsimile serves as the original prescription?

    a. No further documentation is required

    b. A copy of the original prescription must be kept on file

    c. The prescribing practitioner must provide a written confirmation within 72 hours

    d. The dispensing pharmacy must contact the prescribing practitioner for verification

50. What is the primary goal of the DEA's exceptions for facsimile prescriptions of Schedule II controlled substances?

    a. To streamline the prescription process for healthcare providers

    b. To ensure patient safety and access to necessary medications

    c. To reduce the risk of prescription fraud and abuse

    d. To minimize administrative burdens for pharmacies and practitioners

51. What must a pharmacy's electronic system be capable of printing out under the CSA?

    a. Prescribing practitioner's name

    b. Patient's name and address

    c. Quantity and date dispensed on each refill

    d. All of the above

52. How long does the central recordkeeping location have to provide a printout of refill information to a requesting pharmacy?

    a. 24 hours

    b. 48 hours

    c. 72 hours

    d. 96 hours

53. Who has the responsibility to assure that a controlled substance is for a terminally ill patient?

    a. Only the pharmacist

    b. Only the prescribing practitioner

    c. Both the pharmacist and the prescribing practitioner

    d. None of the above

54. What information must the pharmacist record on the prescription for a terminally ill patient?

    a. "Terminally ill"

    b. "LTCF patient"

    c. Both "terminally ill" and "LTCF patient"

    d. None of the above

55. What is required to be included in the refill-by-refill audit trail printout?

    a. Prescribing practitioner's name

    b. Patient's name and address

    c. Quantity and date dispensed on each refill

    d. All of the above

56. How many hours does the prescribing practitioner have to provide a written confirmation for a prescription?

    a. 24 hours

    b. 48 hours

    c. 72 hours

    d. 96 hours

57. What is the maximum number of refills allowed for a controlled substance prescription?

    a. One

    b. Two

    c. Three

    d. Four

58. What is the name or identification code of the dispensing pharmacist required to be included in the refill data printout?

   a. Yes

   b. No

   c. Maybe

   d. Not specified

59. What is the requirement for refills of controlled substances under the CSA?

   a. No refills are allowed

   b. Refills are allowed without any restrictions

   c. The prescribing practitioner must provide a written confirmation within 72 hours

   d. The pharmacist must verify and document the refill data, but no written confirmation is required

60. What is the purpose of maintaining a refill-by-refill audit trail for controlled substances?

   a. To ensure patient safety and access to necessary medications

   b. To track the prescribing practitioner's prescribing patterns

   c. To monitor the pharmacy's inventory of controlled substances

   d. None of the above

61. What is the primary purpose of controlling substances under the law?

    a. To restrict access to certain medications

    b. To ensure proper handling and distribution

    c. To prevent misuse and abuse

    d. All of the above

62. Which government agency is responsible for enforcing controlled substance regulations in the United States?

    a. Food and Drug Administration (FDA)

    b. Drug Enforcement Administration (DEA)

    c. Centers for Disease Control and Prevention (CDC)

    d. National Institutes of Health (NIH)

63. Which schedule of controlled substances includes drugs with the highest potential for abuse and no accepted medical use?

    a. Schedule I

    b. Schedule II

    c. Schedule III

    d. Schedule IV

64. What is the primary difference between Schedule II and Schedule III controlled substances?

   a. Schedule II substances have a higher potential for abuse.

   b. Schedule III substances have a higher potential for abuse.

   c. Schedule II substances have accepted medical uses.

   d. Schedule III substances have accepted medical uses.

65. Which of the following is an example of a Schedule II controlled substance?

   a. Oxycodone

   b. Codeine

   c. Xanax

   d. Ambien

66. What is required for the prescription of Schedule II controlled substances?

   a. A written prescription with no refills

   b. An oral prescription with no refills

   c. A written prescription with refills

   d. An oral prescription with refills

67. Which schedule of controlled substances includes drugs with a moderate to low potential for abuse?

    a. Schedule I

    b. Schedule II

    c. Schedule III

    d. Schedule IV

68. Which of the following is an example of a Schedule III controlled substance?

    a. Heroin

    b. LSD

    c. Ketamine

    d. Anabolic steroids

69. What is required for the prescription of Schedule III controlled substances?

    a. A written prescription with no refills

    b. An oral prescription with no refills

    c. A written prescription with refills

    d. An oral prescription with refills

70. Which schedule of controlled substances includes drugs with the lowest potential for abuse?

    a. Schedule I

    b. Schedule II

    c. Schedule III

    d. Schedule IV

71. Which of the following is an example of a Schedule IV controlled substance?

    a. Heroin

    b. Cocaine

    c. Valium

    d. Methamphetamine

72. What is required for the prescription of Schedule IV controlled substances?

    a. A written prescription with no refills

    b. An oral prescription with no refills

    c. A written prescription with refills

    d. An oral prescription with refills

73. Which schedule of controlled substances includes drugs with a low potential for abuse and accepted medical uses?

    a. Schedule I

    b. Schedule II

    c. Schedule III

    d. Schedule V

74. Which of the following is an example of a Schedule V controlled substance?

    a. Marijuana

    b. LSD

    c. Codeine cough syrup

    d. Ecstasy

75. What is required for the prescription of Schedule V controlled substances?

    a. A written prescription with no refills

    b. An oral prescription with no refills

    c. A written prescription with refills

    d. An oral prescription with refills

76. Which of the following is not a controlled substance?

    a. Alcohol

    b. Nicotine

    c. Caffeine

    d. Aspirin

77. What is the purpose of the Drug Enforcement Administration (DEA) registration?

    a. To track the distribution of controlled substances

    b. To ensure proper handling and storage of controlled substances

    c. To prevent diversion and abuse of controlled substances

    d. All of the above

78. Which of the following is an example of a prescription opioid painkiller?

    a. Ibuprofen

    b. Acetaminophen

    c. Morphine

    d. Naproxen

79. What is the maximum penalty for the illegal possession of a controlled substance?

    a. Fine

    b. Probation

    c. Imprisonment

    d. Community service

80. Which of the following is an example of a commonly abused prescription stimulant?

    a. Ritalin

    b. Prozac

    c. Zoloft

    d. Xanax

81. Which of the following is an example of a Schedule III controlled substance?

    a. Heroin

    b. Cocaine

    c. Vicodin

    d. Methamphetamine

82. What is the maximum penalty for the illegal distribution of a controlled substance?

    a. Fine

    b. Probation

    c. Imprisonment

    d. Community service

83. Which schedule of controlled substances includes drugs with a high potential for abuse and no accepted medical uses?

    a. Schedule I

    b. Schedule II

    c. Schedule III

    d. Schedule IV

84. Which of the following is an example of a Schedule II controlled substance?

    a. Marijuana

    b. LSD

    c. Oxycodone

    d. Xanax

85. What is required for the prescription of Schedule II controlled substances?

    a. A written prescription with no refills

    b. An oral prescription with no refills

    c. A written prescription with refills

    d. An oral prescription with refills

86. Which of the following is an example of a commonly abused prescription opioid?

    a. OxyContin

    b. Prozac

    c. Zoloft

    d. Xanax

87. What is the purpose of the Controlled Substances Act (CSA)?

    a. To regulate the manufacturing and distribution of controlled substances

    b. To classify drugs based on their potential for abuse and medical use

    c. To prevent the illegal use and abuse of controlled substances

    d. All of the above

88. Which of the following is an example of a prescription sedative-hypnotic?

    a. Ibuprofen

    b. Acetaminophen

    c. Ambien

    d. Naproxen

89. What is the maximum penalty for the illegal manufacturing of a controlled substance?

    a. Fine

    b. Probation

    c. Imprisonment

    d. Community service

90. Which of the following is an example of a commonly abused illicit drug?

    a. Heroin

    b. Adderall

    c. Vicodin

    d. OxyContin

91. Which of the following is an example of a Schedule I controlled substance?

    a. Oxycodone

    b. Marijuana

    c. Xanax

    d. Adderall

92. What is the primary purpose of the Drug Enforcement Administration (DEA)?

    a. Regulating over-the-counter medications

    b. Ensuring the safety of dietary supplements

    c. Enforcing controlled substance laws

    d. Monitoring prescription drug prices

93. Which of the following is an example of a Schedule II controlled substance?

    a. Methamphetamine

    b. Valium

    c. Ambien

    d. Tramadol

94. What is required for the prescription of Schedule III controlled substances?

    a. A written prescription with no refills

    b. An oral prescription with no refills

    c. A written prescription with refills

    d. An oral prescription with refills

95. Which of the following is an example of a commonly abused prescription stimulant?

    a. Prozac

    b. Zoloft

    c. Adderall

    d. Xanax

96. Which of the following is an example of a prescription muscle relaxant?

    a. Ibuprofen

    b. Acetaminophen

    c. Flexeril

    d. Naproxen

97. What is the primary purpose of the National Prescription Drug Take Back Day?

    a. To promote the use of prescription drugs

    b. To educate the public about controlled substances

    c. To provide a safe and responsible way to dispose of unused medications

    d. To increase access to controlled substances

98. Which of the following is an example of a Schedule IV controlled substance?

    a. Heroin

    b. Methadone

    c. Xanax

    d. Fentanyl

99. What is the primary factor used to determine the scheduling of a controlled substance?

    a. Potential for abuse

    b. Medical use

    c. Side effects

    d. Cost

100.Which of the following is an example of a commonly abused hallucinogenic drug?

a. Prozac

b. Zoloft

c. LSD

d. Ativan

8.FEDERAL PHARMACY LAW ANSWER PART-8

1. **Answer D**

   Codeine

2. **Answer A**

   Drug Enforcement Administration (DEA)

3. **Answer C**

   Increased heart rate

4. **Answer C**

   Dilated pupils

5. **Answer C**

   Acupuncture

6. **Answer C**

   Increased energy

7. **Answer C**

   Lung damage

8. **Answer D**

   Slowed heart rate

9. **Answer C**

   Increased creativity

10. **Answer D**

    Increased heart rate

11. **Answer C**

    Increased heart rate

12. **Answer D**

    Improved cardiovascular health

13. **Answer D**

    Decreased heart rate

14. **Answer D**

    Weight loss

15. **Answer C**

    Increased sociability

16. **Answer C**

    Increased empathy

17. **Answer D**

    Red eyes

18. Answer A

Liver damage

19. Answer D

Improved sleep quality

20. Answer C

Improved mental health

21. Answer D

Slowed heart rate

22. Answer D

Improved lung function

23. Answer D

Decreased blood pressure

24. Answer C

Liver damage

25. Answer D

Decreased libido

26. Answer D

Improved bone density

27. Answer C

Increased appetite

28. Answer D

Improved cognitive function

29. Answer D

Red eyes

30. Answer A

Liver damage

31. Answer A

Drug Enforcement Administration (DEA)

32. Answer A

Schedule I

33. Answer B

Accepted medical use

34. Answer A

Controlled Substances Act (CSA)

35. Answer D

Public apology

36. Answer D

Mandatory drug rehabilitation

37. Answer D

Public warning

38. Answer D

Community service

39. Answer C

Mandatory drug testing

40. Answer D

Increased insurance premiums

41. Answer B

DEA

42. Answer D

All of the above

43. Answer D

All of the above

44. Answer D

All healthcare facilities

45. Answer D

All of the above

46. Answer C

Three

47. Answer D

All of the above

48. Answer A

No refills are allowed

49. Answer C

The prescribing practitioner must provide a written confirmation within 72 hours

50. Answer B

To ensure patient safety and access to necessary medications

51. Answer D

All of the above

52. Answer B

48 hours

53. Answer C

Both the pharmacist and the prescribing practitioner

54. Answer C

Both "terminally ill" and "LTCF patient"

55. Answer D

All of the above

56. Answer C

72 hours

57. Answer C

Three

58. Answer B

No

59. Answer C

The prescribing practitioner must provide a written confirmation within 72 hours

60. Answer A

To ensure patient safety and access to necessary medications

61. Answer D

All of the above

62. Answer B

Drug Enforcement Administration (DEA)

63. Answer A

Schedule I

64. Answer C

Schedule II substances have accepted medical uses.

65. Answer A

Oxycodone

66. Answer A

A written prescription with no refills

67. Answer C

Schedule III

68. Answer D

Anabolic steroids

69. Answer C

A written prescription with refills

70. Answer D

Schedule IV

71. Answer C

Valium

72. Answer C

A written prescription with refills

73. Answer D

Schedule V

74. Answer C

Codeine cough syrup

75. Answer C

A written prescription with refills

76. Answer D

Aspirin

77. Answer D

All of the above

78. Answer C

Morphine

79. Answer C

Imprisonment

80. Answer A

Ritalin

81. Answer C

Vicodin

82. Answer C

Imprisonment

83. Answer A

Schedule I

84. Answer C

Oxycodone

85. Answer A

A written prescription with no refills

86. Answer A

OxyContin

87. Answer D

All of the above

88. Answer C

Ambien

89. Answer C

Imprisonment

90. Answer A

Heroin

91. Answer B

Marijuana

92. Answer C

Enforcing controlled substance laws

93. Answer A

Methamphetamine

94. Answer C

A written prescription with refills

95. Answer C

Adderall

96. Answer C

Flexeril

97. Answer C

To provide a safe and responsible way to dispose of unused medications

98. Answer C

Xanax

99. Answer A

Potential for abuse

100. Answer C

LSD

9. FEDERAL PHARMACY LAW QUESTION PART-9

1. What is the primary responsibility of a pharmacist?

    a. Dispensing medication

    b. Providing medical advice

    c. Managing inventory

    d. Billing insurance companies

2. Which of the following is a duty of a pharmacist?

    a. Diagnosing medical conditions

    b. Administering vaccines

    c. Prescribing medication

    d. Monitoring drug interactions

3. What is the role of a pharmacist in patient care?

    a. Providing emotional support

    b. Monitoring medication adherence

    c. Conducting physical exams

    d. Creating treatment plans

4. What is the responsibility of a pharmacist in ensuring medication safety?

   a. Checking for drug interactions

   b. Writing prescriptions

   c. Managing patient records

   d. Performing surgeries

5. Which of the following is a duty of a pharmacist in managing medication inventory?

   a. Ordering supplies

   b. Cleaning equipment

   c. Conducting clinical trials

   d. Providing patient education

6. What is the responsibility of a pharmacist in managing controlled substances?

   a. Administering medication

   b. Ensuring compliance with regulations

   c. Providing emergency care

   d. Conducting research studies

7. Which of the following is a duty of a pharmacist in providing patient education?

    a. Monitoring vital signs

    b. Explaining medication instructions

    c. Conducting physical therapy

    d. Performing laboratory tests

8. What is the role of a pharmacist in preventing medication errors?

    a. Providing counseling services

    b. Checking prescriptions for accuracy

    c. Conducting medical procedures

    d. Managing patient billing

9. Which of the following is a responsibility of a pharmacist in managing drug interactions?

    a. Prescribing medication

    b. Monitoring side effects

    c. Performing surgeries

    d. Conducting physical exams

10. What is the duty of a pharmacist in ensuring medication adherence?

    a. Monitoring vital signs

    b. Providing medication reminders

    c. Conducting laboratory tests

    d. Administering vaccines

11. Which of the following is a responsibility of a pharmacist in managing drug allergies?

    a. Prescribing medication

    b. Providing counseling services

    c. Conducting physical exams

    d. Monitoring medication interactions

12. What is the role of a pharmacist in managing medication dosage?

    a. Prescribing medication

    b. Monitoring side effects

    c. Providing medication education

    d. Conducting medical procedures

13. Which of the following is a duty of a pharmacist in managing medication side effects?

    a. Providing emotional support

    b. Adjusting medication dosage

    c. Conducting laboratory tests

    d. Administering vaccines

14. What is the responsibility of a pharmacist in managing medication storage?

    a. Ordering supplies

    b. Cleaning equipment

    c. Ensuring proper temperature control

    d. Conducting clinical trials

15. Which of the following is a duty of a pharmacist in providing medication counseling?

    a. Monitoring vital signs

    b. Explaining medication instructions

    c. Performing physical therapy

    d. Conducting research studies

16. What is the role of a pharmacist in managing medication interactions with food and drink?

    a. Prescribing medication

    b. Monitoring side effects

    c. Providing dietary advice

    d. Conducting medical procedures

17. Which of the following is a responsibility of a pharmacist in managing medication contraindications?

    a. Prescribing medication

    b. Monitoring side effects

    c. Providing counseling services

    d. Conducting physical exams

18. What is the duty of a pharmacist in managing medication expiration dates?

    a. Ordering supplies

    b. Cleaning equipment

    c. Ensuring proper disposal

    d. Conducting clinical trials

19. Which of the following is a responsibility of a pharmacist in managing medication interactions with other medical conditions?

    a. Prescribing medication

    b. Monitoring side effects

    c. Providing counseling services

    d. Conducting physical exams

20. What is the role of a pharmacist in managing medication interactions with other medications?

    a. Prescribing medication

    b. Monitoring side effects

    c. Providing counseling services

    d. Conducting research studies

21. What is the primary responsibility of a pharmacist?

    a. Dispensing medication

    b. Providing medical advice

    c. Conducting clinical trials

    d. Performing surgery

22. What is the duty of a pharmacist in ensuring patient safety?

    a. Prescribing medication

    b. Monitoring drug interactions

    c. Conducting physical exams

    d. Administering vaccines

23. What is the role of a pharmacist in managing chronic diseases?

    a. Providing counseling on lifestyle changes

    b. Performing surgeries

    c. Prescribing medication

    d. Providing emergency care

24. What is the duty of a pharmacist in ensuring medication adherence?

    a. Providing medication reminders

    b. Dispensing medication only

    c. Conducting physical exams

    d. Performing lab tests

25. What is the responsibility of a pharmacist in managing drug inventory?

    a. Ordering and stocking medication

    b. Conducting clinical trials

    c. Providing medical advice

    d. Administering vaccines

26. What is the role of a pharmacist in providing immunization services?

    a. Dispensing medication only

    b. Administering vaccines

    c. Providing medical advice

    d. Conducting physical exams

27. What is the duty of a pharmacist in managing drug interactions?

    a. Providing counseling on lifestyle changes

    b. Prescribing medication

    c. Monitoring drug interactions

    d. Performing surgeries

28. What is the responsibility of a pharmacist in providing medication therapy management?

    a. Dispensing medication only

    b. Monitoring drug interactions

    c. Conducting physical exams

    d. Providing counseling on medication use

29. What is the role of a pharmacist in providing patient education?

    a. Prescribing medication

    b. Providing medical advice

    c. Dispensing medication only

    d. Counseling on medication use and side effects

30. What is the duty of a pharmacist in ensuring medication safety?

    a. Providing medical advice

    b. Dispensing medication only

    c. Monitoring for adverse drug reactions

    d. Conducting physical exams

31. What is the primary role of a pharmacist when dispensing a drug?

    a. Providing patient counseling

    b. Administering injections

    c. Conducting medical examinations

    d. Performing surgical procedures

32. Which of the following is a key step in the drug dispensing process?

    a. Patient diagnosis

    b. Prescription verification

    c. Medical billing

    d. General inventory management

33. Pharmacist plays a vital role in:

    a. Diagnosing medical conditions

    b. Monitoring patient vital signs

    c. Safety and accuracy of drug dispensing

    d. Conducting surgical procedures

34. In the context of medication dispensing, what does the term "compounding" refer to?

    a. Mixing ingredients to prepare personalized medications

    b. Administering medications to patients

    c. Discarding expired medications

    d. Performing drug interactions analysis

35. Which of the following is an essential task in drug dispensing performed by pharmacists?

    a. Setting drug prices

    b. Conducting medical research

    c. Providing patient education

    d. Performing surgical procedures

36. What should a pharmacist verify before dispensing a drug to a patient?

    a. Patient diagnosis

    b. Prescriber's credentials

    c. Medication cost

    d. Patient's food allergies

37. What type of regulations are pharmacists required to comply with?

    a. International travel guidelines

    b. Tax preparation regulations

    c. Pharmacy accreditation standards

    d. Banking laws and regulations

38. Which government agency oversees the regulations for pharmacists?

    a. National Aeronautics and Space Administration (NASA)

    b. Food and Drug Administration (FDA)

    c. Federal Communications Commission (FCC)

    d. Department of Homeland Security (DHS)

39. What is the purpose of the Drug Enforcement Administration (DEA) in relation to pharmacists?

    a. Ensuring safe handling and distribution of controlled substances

    b. Overseeing pharmacist licensure exams

    c. Managing healthcare facilities' budget allocations

    d. Establishing medication pricing guidelines

40. What should pharmacists do if they encounter a questionable prescription?

    a. Dispense the medication without further inquiry

    b. Contact the prescribing doctor for clarification

    c. Refuse to dispense the medication without providing any explanation

    d. Ask the patient to switch to an over-the-counter alternative

41. What does HIPAA stand for in the realm of pharmacy practice?

    a. Health Insurance Portability and Accountability Act

    b. Healthcare Industry Privacy and Accountability Act

    c. Hospital Insurance Provision and Accessibility Act

    d. Health Records Processing and Authorization Act

42. Pharmacists are responsible for monitoring potential drug interactions. How is this typically accomplished?

    a. Utilizing computerized drug interaction checking systems

    b. Assigning a clinical pharmacist to each patient

    c. Conducting regular patient follow-up visits

    d. Relying solely on the prescriber's expertise

43. Which of the following is an example of a prescription-only medication?

    a. Over-the-counter pain reliever

    b. Antibacterial hand sanitizer

    c. Insulin for diabetes treatment

    d. Cough drops

44. Which organization ensures that a pharmacist's education meets minimum standards?

    a. World Health Organization (WHO)

    b. National Association of Boards of Pharmacy (NABP)

    c. American Medical Association (AMA)

    d. United Nations (UN)

45. In order to prevent medication errors, pharmacists should:

    a. Double-check the prescriptions against the patient's medical history

    b. Dispense medications without verifying the package seals

    c. Trust the prescriber's instructions completely

    d. Avoid employing pharmacy technicians

46. What is a medication therapy management service provided by pharmacists?

    a. Counseling patients on general health and wellness

    b. Performing cosmetic procedures

    c. Administering vaccinations

    d. Collaborating with other healthcare providers to optimize medication therapy

47. How often can a Schedule II controlled substance be dispensed?

    a. Once every 30 days

    b. Once every 60 days

    c. Once every 90 days

    d. Once every 180 days

48. How often can a Schedule III or IV controlled substance be dispensed?

    a. Once every 30 days

    b. Once every 60 days

    c. Once every 90 days

    d. Once every 180 days

49. How often can a Schedule V controlled substance be dispensed?

    a. Once every 30 days

    b. Once every 60 days

    c. Once every 90 days

    d. Once every 180 days

50. How does a pharmacist dispense a drug?

    a. By counting pills and packaging them

    b. By mixing ingredients and preparing a compound

    c. By providing counseling and education to patients

    d. By administering injections or infusions

51. What is the role of a pharmacist in the dispensing process?

    a. To prescribe medications to patients

    b. To verify the accuracy of the prescription

    c. To administer medications to patients

    d. To conduct clinical trials for new drugs

52. How does a pharmacist ensure the safety of the dispensed drug?

    a. By checking for drug interactions and allergies

    b. By sterilizing the medication before dispensing

    c. By conducting laboratory tests on the drug

    d. By providing a detailed medication guide to the patient

53. How does a pharmacist handle controlled substances?

    a. By storing them in a secure area and maintaining accurate records

    b. By dispensing them without any special precautions

    c. By diluting them to reduce their potency

    d. By disposing of them in regular trash bins

54. What is the purpose of prescription labeling by a pharmacist?

    a. To provide instructions for taking the medication

    b. To indicate the expiration date of the medication

    c. To list potential side effects of the medication

    d. To identify the manufacturer of the medication

55. How does a pharmacist handle medication errors?

    a. By reporting them to the prescriber and documenting the incident

    b. By ignoring them if they are minor in nature

    c. By blaming the patient for the error

    d. By discarding the medication and starting over

56. How does a pharmacist ensure patient confidentiality?

    a. By maintaining secure electronic health records

    b. By discussing patient information openly with others

    c. By selling patient information to third parties

    d. By posting patient information on social media platforms

57. How often can a Schedule II controlled substance be dispensed for a patient with chronic pain?

    a. Once every 30 days

    b. Once every 60 days

    c. Once every 90 days

    d. Once every 180 days

58. How often can a Schedule III or IV controlled substance be dispensed for a patient with acute pain?

   a. Once every 30 days

   b. Once every 60 days

   c. Once every 90 days

   d. Once every 180 days

59. How often can a Schedule V controlled substance be dispensed for a patient with a seizure disorder?

   a. Once every 30 days

   b. Once every 60 days

   c. Once every 90 days

   d. Once every 180 days

60. How does a pharmacist ensure the accuracy of a dispensed drug?

   a. By using automated dispensing systems

   b. By double-checking the prescription with another pharmacist

   c. By conducting regular audits of the dispensing process

   d. By relying on the manufacturer's quality control

61. What is the role of a pharmacist in medication therapy management?

    a. To monitor patients for adverse drug reactions

    b. To adjust medication dosages based on patient response

    c. To collaborate with healthcare providers to optimize therapy

    d. All of the above

62. How does a pharmacist handle drug recalls?

    a. By notifying patients and providing alternative medications

    b. By ignoring the recall and continuing to dispense the drug

    c. By returning the recalled drug to the manufacturer for a refund

    d. By selling the recalled drug at a discounted price

63. How does a pharmacist handle medication shortages?

    a. By working with healthcare providers to find suitable alternatives

    b. By rationing the available medication to patients

    c. By increasing the price of the medication due to scarcity

    d. By refusing to dispense any medication during a shortage

64. How does a pharmacist ensure the proper storage of medications?

    a. By maintaining appropriate temperature and humidity conditions

    b. By storing medications in a locked cabinet to prevent theft

    c. By regularly inspecting the storage area for expired medications

    d. All of the above

65. How does a pharmacist handle medication non-adherence by a patient?

    a. By providing counseling and education to improve adherence

    b. By refusing to refill the medication until the patient complies

    c. By reporting the patient to law enforcement for non-compliance

    d. By increasing the dosage of the medication to compensate for non-adherence

66. How does a pharmacist contribute to patient safety in the dispensing process?

    a. By conducting medication reconciliation to prevent drug interactions

    b. By verifying the patient's identity before dispensing the medication

    c. By providing clear instructions for taking the medication

    d. All of the above

67. What kind of regulations govern the licensing and registration of pharmacists?

    a. State pharmacy practice acts

    b. Federal Controlled Substances Act

    c. Occupational Safety and Health Administration (OSHA) regulations

    d. Food and Drug Administration (FDA) regulations

68. What kind of regulations govern the handling and storage of controlled substances by a pharmacist?

    a. Drug Enforcement Administration (DEA) regulations

    b. Health Insurance Portability and Accountability Act (HIPAA) regulations

    c. Federal Food, Drug, and Cosmetic Act (FD&C Act)

    d. Americans with Disabilities Act (ADA)

69. What kind of regulations govern the labeling and packaging of medications by a pharmacist?

    a. Federal Poison Prevention Packaging Act (PPPA)

    b. Occupational Safety and Health Administration (OSHA) regulations

    c. Health Insurance Portability and Accountability Act (HIPAA) regulations

    d. Americans with Disabilities Act (ADA)

70. What kind of regulations govern the compounding of medications by a pharmacist?

    a. United States Pharmacopeia (USP) standards

    b. Federal Controlled Substances Act

    c. Federal Food, Drug, and Cosmetic Act (FD&C Act)

    d. Occupational Safety and Health Administration (OSHA) regulations

71. What kind of regulations govern the reporting of adverse drug reactions by a pharmacist?

    a. Med Watch reporting requirements

    b. Health Insurance Portability and Accountability Act (HIPAA) regulations

    c. Federal Poison Prevention Packaging Act (PPPA)

    d. Americans with Disabilities Act (ADA)

72. What kind of regulations govern the dispensing of medications to minors by a pharmacist?

    a. State laws regarding the age of consent for medical treatment

    b. Federal Controlled Substances Act

    c. United States Pharmacopeia (USP) standards

    d. Occupational Safety and Health Administration (OSHA) regulations

73. What kind of regulations govern the counseling of patients by a pharmacist?

    a. State pharmacy practice acts

    b. Federal Food, Drug, and Cosmetic Act (FD&C Act)

    c. Health Insurance Portability and Accountability Act (HIPAA) regulations

    d. Americans with Disabilities Act (ADA)

74. What kind of regulations govern the documentation and record-keeping by a pharmacist?

    a. Health Insurance Portability and Accountability Act (HIPAA) regulations

    b. Federal Controlled Substances Act

    c. Occupational Safety and Health Administration (OSHA) regulations

    d. State pharmacy practice acts

75. What kind of regulations govern the disposal of medications by a pharmacist?

    a. Drug Enforcement Administration (DEA) regulations

    b. Federal Poison Prevention Packaging Act (PPPA)

    c. United States Pharmacopeia (USP) standards

    d. Americans with Disabilities Act (ADA)

76. What kind of regulations govern the advertising and promotion of medications by a pharmacist?

    a. Federal Food, Drug, and Cosmetic Act (FD&C Act)

    b. Health Insurance Portability and Accountability Act (HIPAA) regulations

    c. Occupational Safety and Health Administration (OSHA) regulations

    d. State pharmacy practice acts

77. What is the first step a pharmacist takes when dispensing a drug?

    a. Check the prescription label

    b. Verify the patient's identity

    c. Count the pills

    d. None of the above

78. What is the purpose of a pharmacist's counseling session with a patient?

    a. To explain how to take the medication

    b. To answer any questions about the medication

    c. To discuss potential side effects

    d. All of the above

79. How does a pharmacist ensure the safety of a medication?

    a. By checking for drug interactions

    b. By verifying the dosage and strength

    c. By checking for allergies

    d. All of the above

80. What is the role of a pharmacist in ensuring medication adherence?

    a. To educate patients on the importance of taking their medication as prescribed

    b. To monitor patients' medication use and refill history

    c. To provide medication reminders

    d. All of the above

81. What is the purpose of a medication label?

    a. To provide information about the medication

    b. To ensure proper dosing and administration

    c. To prevent medication errors

    d. All of the above

82. How does a pharmacist handle a medication that has been recalled?

    a. Remove the medication from inventory and notify patients who received it

    b. Continue to dispense the medication until further notice

    c. Wait for further instructions from the manufacturer

    d. None of the above

83. What is the pharmacist's role in preventing medication errors?

    a. To check for drug interactions

    b. To verify the dosage and strength

    c. To ensure proper labeling and packaging

    d. All of the above

84. How does a pharmacist handle a medication that has expired?

    a. Remove the medication from inventory and dispose of it properly

    b. Continue to dispense the medication until it runs out

    c. Wait for further instructions from the manufacturer

    d. None of the above

85. What is the process for dispensing a controlled substance?

    a. Verify the prescriber's DEA number

    b. Verify the patient's identity

    c. Verify the prescription's authenticity

    d. All of the above

86. What is the role of a pharmacist in managing drug therapy?

    a. To monitor patients' medication use and refill history

    b. To adjust medication doses as needed

    c. To provide medication counseling

    d. All of the above

87. What is the purpose of a medication reconciliation?

    a. To ensure accurate medication records

    b. To identify potential drug interactions

    c. To prevent medication errors

    d. All of the above

88. How does a pharmacist handle a medication that has been tampered with?

    a. Remove the medication from inventory and notify patients who received it

    b. Continue to dispense the medication until further notice

    c. Wait for further instructions from the manufacturer

    d. None of the above

89. What is the role of a pharmacist in ensuring medication safety during pregnancy?

    a. To counsel pregnant patients on medication risks and benefits

    b. To monitor medication use during pregnancy

    c. To adjust medication doses as needed

    d. All of the above

90. What is the process for handling a medication recall?

    a. Remove the medication from inventory and notify patients who received it

    b. Wait for further instructions from the manufacturer

    c. Continue to dispense the medication until further notice

    d. None of the above

91. What is the role of a pharmacist in managing medication-related adverse events?

    a. To monitor patients for adverse events

    b. To report adverse events to the appropriate authorities

    c. To adjust medication doses as needed

    d. All of the above

92. What is the pharmacist's role in ensuring medication safety for pediatric patients?

    a. To counsel parents on medication risks and benefits

    b. To adjust medication doses based on age and weight

    c. To monitor medication use in pediatric patients

    d. All of the above

93. Which of the following is a duty of a pharmacist?

    a. Dispensing medication

    b. Performing surgery

    c. Conducting medical exams

    d. Providing legal advice

94. What is the responsibility of a pharmacist?

   a. Diagnosing medical conditions

   b. Monitoring medication adherence

   c. Performing physical therapy

   d. Conducting surgical procedures

95. Which of the following is a duty of a pharmacist?

   a. Delivering babies

   b. Monitoring drug interactions

   c. Performing dental procedures

   d. Conducting psychological evaluations

96. Which of the following is a duty of a pharmacist?

   a. Repairing medical equipment

   b. Ordering supplies

   c. Conducting x-rays

   d. Providing legal representation

97. What is the responsibility of a pharmacist?

    a. Prescribing medication

    b. Ensuring compliance with regulations

    c. Performing surgery

    d. Conducting physical exams

98. Which of the following is a duty of a pharmacist?

    a. Providing dental care

    b. Explaining medication instructions

    c. Conducting chiropractic adjustments

    d. Performing cosmetic surgery

99. What is the responsibility of a pharmacist?

    a. Checking for dental cavities

    b. Checking prescriptions for accuracy

    c. Conducting vision tests

    d. Providing tax advice

100. What is the responsibility of a pharmacist?

a. Providing legal representation

b. Monitoring side effects

c. Conducting brain scans

d. Prescribing medication without a doctor's approval

9. FEDERAL PHARMACY LAW ANSWER PART-9

1. **Answer A**

   Dispensing medication

2. **Answer D**

   Monitoring drug interactions

3. **Answer B**

   Monitoring medication adherence

4. **Answer A**

   Checking for drug interactions

5. **Answer A**

   Ordering supplies

6. **Answer B**

   Ensuring compliance with regulations

7. **Answer B**

   Explaining medication instructions

8. **Answer B**

   Checking prescriptions for accuracy

9. **Answer B**

Monitoring side effects

10. **Answer B**

Providing medication reminders

11. **Answer D**

Monitoring medication interactions

12. **Answer B**

Monitoring side effects

13. **Answer B**

Adjusting medication dosage

14. **Answer C**

Ensuring proper temperature control

15. **Answer B**

Explaining medication instructions

16. **Answer C**

Providing dietary advice

17. **Answer C**

Providing counseling services

18. **Answer C**

Ensuring proper disposal

19. **Answer C**

Providing counseling services

20. **Answer B**

Monitoring side effects

21. **Answer A**

Dispensing medication

22. **Answer B**

Monitoring drug interactions

23. **Answer A**

Providing counseling on lifestyle changes

24. **Answer A**

Providing medication reminders

25. **Answer A**

Ordering and stocking medication

26. **Answer B**

Administering vaccines

27. Answer C

Monitoring drug interactions

28. Answer D

Providing counseling on medication use

29. Answer D

Counseling on medication use and side effects

30. Answer C

Monitoring for adverse drug reactions

31. Answer A

Providing patient counseling

32. Answer B

Prescription verification

33. Answer C

Safety and accuracy of drug dispensing

34. Answer A

Mixing ingredients to prepare personalized medications

35. Answer C

Providing patient education

36. Answer B

Prescriber's credentials

37. Answer C

Pharmacy accreditation standards

38. Answer B

Food and Drug Administration (FDA)

39. Answer A

Ensuring safe handling and distribution of controlled substances

40. Answer B

Contact the prescribing doctor for clarification

41. Answer A

Health Insurance Portability and Accountability Act

42. Answer A

Utilizing computerized drug interaction checking systems

43. Answer C

Insulin for diabetes treatment

44. Answer B

National Association of Boards of Pharmacy (NABP)

45. Answer A

Double-check the prescriptions against the patient's medical history

46. Answer D

Collaborating with other healthcare providers to optimize medication therapy

47. Answer A

Once every 30 days

48. Answer C

Once every 90 days

49. Answer C

Once every 90 days

50. Answer A

By counting pills and packaging them

51. Answer B

To verify the accuracy of the prescription

52. Answer A

By checking for drug interactions and allergies

53. Answer A

By storing them in a secure area and maintaining accurate records

54. Answer A

To provide instructions for taking the medication

55. Answer A

By reporting them to the prescriber and documenting the incident

56. Answer A

By maintaining secure electronic health records

57. Answer A

Once every 30 days

58. Answer A

Once every 30 days

59. Answer A

Once every 30 days

60. Answer B

By double-checking the prescription with another pharmacist

61. Answer D

All of the above

62. Answer A

By notifying patients and providing alternative medications

63. Answer A

By working with healthcare providers to find suitable alternatives

64. Answer D

All of the above

65. Answer A

By providing counseling and education to improve adherence

66. Answer D

All of the above

67. Answer A

State pharmacy practice acts

68. Answer A

Drug Enforcement Administration (DEA) regulations

69. Answer A

Federal Poison Prevention Packaging Act (PPPA)

70. Answer A

United States Pharmacopeia (USP) standards

71. Answer A

Med Watch reporting requirements

72. Answer A

State laws regarding the age of consent for medical treatment

73. Answer A

State pharmacy practice acts

74. Answer D

State pharmacy practice acts

75. Answer A

Drug Enforcement Administration (DEA) regulations

76. Answer A

Federal Food, Drug, and Cosmetic Act (FD&C Act)

77. Answer A

Check the prescription label

78. Answer D

All of the above

79. Answer D

All of the above

80. Answer D

All of the above

81. Answer D

All of the above

82. Answer A

Remove the medication from inventory and notify patients who received it

83. Answer D

All of the above

84. Answer A

Remove the medication from inventory and dispose of it properly

85. Answer D

All of the above

86. Answer D

All of the above

87. Answer D

All of the above

88. Answer A

Remove the medication from inventory and notify patients who received it

89. Answer D

All of the above

90. Answer A

Remove the medication from inventory and notify patients who received it

91. Answer D

All of the above

92. Answer D

All of the above

93. Answer A

Dispensing medication

94. Answer B

Monitoring medication adherence

95. Answer B

Monitoring drug interactions

96. Answer B

Ordering supplies

97. Answer B

Ensuring compliance with regulations

98. Answer B

Explaining medication instructions

99. Answer B

Checking prescriptions for accuracy

100. Answer B

Monitoring side effects

www.ingramcontent.com/pod-product-compliance
Lightning Source LLC
Chambersburg PA
CBHW062347220526
45472CB00008B/1723
* 9 7 9 8 3 0 0 7 3 1 3 8 0 *